# Peritoneal Dialysis

*Vlatko Karanfilovski*
*Pavlina Dzekova-Vidimliski*

Title: Peritoneal Dialysis

ISBN: 979-8-89248-572-2

Author: Vlatko Karanfilovski, Pavlina Dzekova-Vidimliski

Cover image: https://pixabay.com/

Publisher: Generis Publishing
Online orders: www.generis-publishing.com
Contact email: info@generis-publishing.com

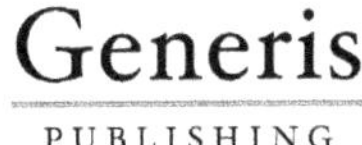

# Table of contents

# Peritoneal dialysis – summary

Kidney failure (KF) is characterized by a severe decrease in kidney function with a glomerular filtration rate (GFR) of less than 15mL/min/1.73 m$^2$ with a need to start treatment with kidney replacement therapy (KRT). The modalities of KRT are peritoneal dialysis (PD), hemodialysis, and kidney transplantation. Peritoneal dialysis (PD) is a high-quality, cost-effective, home-based dialysis modality. The percentage of patients with kidney failure treated with PD was 5%-10% in economically developed regions like the United States and Western Europe. A percentage of 75% was registered in Mexico, where PD was the first choice for KRT, due to the higher costs of hemodialysis and difficulty accessing a hemodialysis unit.

In PD, the peritoneal membrane is used as a dialyzing surface that provides an exchange of solutes and fluid between the peritoneal capillary blood and the dialysis solution that is instilled into the peritoneal cavity. During this process, based on the concentration gradient, solutes such as urea, creatinine, and potassium diffuse from the peritoneal capillaries across the peritoneal membrane to dialysis solution in the peritoneal cavity. The hyperosmolality of the dialysis solution achieved by adding a different concentration of dextrose allows the removal of excess water from the blood to the dialysis solution through the process of osmosis. The access for peritoneal dialysis is a catheter inserted into the peritoneal cavity. PD could be performed either manually as in continuous ambulatory peritoneal dialysis (CAPD) or by using a PD machine as in automated PD (APD).

Despite the treatment practice and technical improvements in PD over the past decade, PD-related peritonitis remains the major complication. The non-infectious PD complications are abdominal wall–related hernias, leakages of dialysis fluid, and malfunction of the PD catheter.

The epidemiology of PD, PD techniques, basic principles of PD prescription, monitoring of PD adequacy, and PD-related complications were described in the book. The treatment of anemia, mineral bone disease, nutrition in PD patients, and the prescription of PD in cases of pandemics and natural disasters were also discussed in the book.

*Chapter 1*

*Modalities of kidney replacement therapy: dialysis and transplantation.
History of peritoneal dialysis*

Patients with chronic kidney disease stage 5 (kidney failure) require treatment with kidney replacement therapy (KRT). KRT includes treatment with dialysis (hemodialysis or peritoneal dialysis) and kidney transplantation. Hemodialysis (HD) can be delivered at home, in special centers for dialysis, or in a hospital. Peritoneal dialysis is done at home and can be continuous ambulatory PD (CAPD) or automated PD (APD). Kidney transplantation may be pre-emptive (before dialysis) or done after starting treatment with dialysis. The kidney for transplantation may be from a living or deceased donor. For feasible patients with kidney failure, receiving a functioning kidney transplant offers substantial lifestyle advantages compared to maintenance dialysis (hemodialysis or peritoneal dialysis). These advantages are partly counterbalanced by the short-term surgical risks and long-term medical risks (infections and malignancies) from immunosuppression. However, many studies have demonstrated that patients who received kidney transplants had a longer life expectancy and better quality of life than those with equivalent health status who were on maintenance dialysis. The waiting lists for kidney transplant are usually long and not every patient is feasible for transplantation, so maintenance dialysis (PD and/or HD) remains the commonest form of KRT for patients with kidney failure.

## 1.1.  Hemodialysis and peritoneal dialysis

The patients treated with HD or PD need to do some adaptation to the treatment modality and lifestyle modifications. High-flow vascular access must be created in patients treated with HD. Hemodialysis treatment usually is delivered in medical units-centers for hemodialysis, thrice time per week, approximately 4 hours per dialysis session. However, some variations in the location, length, or frequency of each dialysis session are possible: In - center hemodialysis or home hemodialysis (thrice time per week, approximately 4 hours per dialysis session).

- Frequent short daily HD of 2.5 to 3 hours per session or long thrice weekly HD sessions of 5 to 7 hours each.
- Nocturnal home or in-center long-duration HD.

These alternative hemodialysis regiments (higher frequency and/or longer duration of the HD sessions) have shown better effects on reductions in blood pressure and the use of antihypertensive medications, reduction of serum phosphorus levels, with smaller changes in left ventricular mass (LV hypertrophy), and risk of death. Moreover, patients treated with nocturnal HD appeared to have similar outcomes as patients with transplanted kidney from deceased donor.

Peritoneal dialysis is done at home, and there are two PD modalities: continuous ambulatory PD (CAPD) and automated PD (APD). In most developed countries, APD has become a dominant PD modality with a significant positive impact on patients' lives. In developing world and emerging economies, CAPD remains the predominant PD modality. Available data from a few studies failed to show significant differences in medical outcomes in patients treated with CAPD and APD. Hence, economic considerations remained the major determinant in the choice between these two PD modalities.

The comparison of the outcomes between patients treated with HD and PD was difficult and with limited validity. Usually, patients had a preference for one modality and refused to be randomized. Few smaller studies demonstrated early survival advantage (lower risk of death in the first two years for patients on PD) but it was unclear whether this was a direct benefit of the dialysis modality or it was secondary to a higher risk of death among patients who started HD with central venous catheter.

Economic evaluation of dialysis treatment had shown that home-based therapies (PD and home HD) were less expensive than in-center hemodialysis. Moreover, the use of these modalities offered significant cost savings with improvement in the quality of life of the patients at the same time.

In the majority of the KF patients there were no compelling medical reasons to choose one particular dialysis therapy and only a minority of patients have clear medical advantages in choosing PD instead of HD and vice versa. Hence, the patients should be properly educated on all modalities of KRT, to choose the modality that allows them the most productive and quality life.


## 1.2.  History of peritoneal dialysis

The concept of peritoneal dialysis as a modality of KRT is a hundred years old. The PD solutions and PD technique have evolved to the achievement of today's form.

There is a short review of the milestones in PD history, starting from its origins to the present day:

- **Rene Dutrochet (1776-1846):** introduced the term "osmosis" which explains ultrafiltration in peritoneal dialysis.
- **Thomas Graham (1805-1869):** has done **a** precise description of the osmotic forces of fluids and the difference between crystalloids and colloids.
- **Christopher Warrick, a surgeon from Truro in England (early 19<sup>th</sup> century):** presented a drastic method of treating recurrent ascites: He managed a female patient aged 50 with severe ascites by infusing a mixture of one-half bristol water and one-half claret into the peritoneal cavity after draining the ascites. He believed that ascites is a consequence of rupture of abdominal lymphatics and looked for a method to close them.
- **Recklinghausen, Wegner, Beck, and Kollossow (later half of the 19th century):** described the mesothelium, transport of solutes and water across the peritoneum, and also described the pathways of transport.
- **Bobb et al. (late 19<sup>th</sup> century):** described the "bi-directional permeability" of the peritoneal membrane (blood to peritoneal cavity and vice versa).
- **Starling and Tubby (1894):** theories and physiological explanations for the solute transport between the peritoneal cavity and blood (Starling's forces).
- **Georg Ganter (1923):** the first article on the use of peritoneal cavity in experimental uremia in guinea pigs – **first peritoneal dialysis.** The findings were published in his paper "On the elimination of toxic substances from the blood by dialysis".
- **Arnold Seligman, Jacob Fine, and Howard Frank (1945):** treated patient with acute kidney failure due to sulpha overdose with PD.
- **Northon Maxwell (1959):** simplified the technique.
- **Boen (Seattle, 1962):**
  - First long term PD programmed,
  - First automated PD machine,
  - Explain diffusion curve, peritoneal clearance, and the influence of glucose on ultrafiltration,
  - Added bicarbonate to the fluid to correct acidosis,
  - Developed a close system to limit the risk of infections.
- **Tenckhoff (1968):** developed the revolutionary "Tenckhoff catheter" for PD that changed the PD practice worldwide.
- **Moncreif and Popovic (Austin, Texas; 1975):** initiated patients on continuous mode of PD and named it CAPD.

- **Umberto Buoncristiani (Italy; 1980):** developed the most accepted modern form of CAPD. He introduced the "Y-set" and the "flash before fill" which reduced the incidence of peritonitis.
- **Bazzato (1980):** Double bag system.
- **Diaz-Buxo (1981):** developed APD/CCPD.

## References


1. Deepa C, Muralidhar K. Renal replacement therapy in ICU. J Anaesthesiol Clin Pharmacol. 2012 Jul;28(3):386-396.
2. Lobo VA. Renal Replacement Therapy in Acute Kidney Injury: Which Mode and When? Indian J Crit Care Med. 2020 Apr;24(Suppl 3): S102-S106.
3. Mehrota R, Kalantar-Zedeh K. . Outcomes of kidney replacement therapies. In: Scott J. Gilbert and Daniel E. Weiner. Primer of kidney diseases. Elsevier 2014; Sixth edition:534-541.
4. National Institute for Health and Care Excellence. RRT and conservative management - Modalities of RRT. NICE guideline NG107, Evidence Review, October 2018.
5. Oreopoulos, D.G. and Thodis, E. The history of peritoneal dialysis: Early years at Toronto Western Hospital. Dial.Transplant. 2010; 39:338-343.
6. Agarwal S, Wilkie M. Remote Patient Management in Peritoneal Dialysis: Opportunities and Challenges. Contrib Nephrol. 2019; 197:54-64.

## Chapter 2
## *Epidemiology of peritoneal dialysis*

A systemic review of data from 123 countries (representing 93% of the world's population) estimated that 2.618 million people received KRT worldwide in 2010 and this number would be doubled to 5.439 million people by the year 2030, with the highest growth in low-income and middle-income countries (Asia and Latin America). As the global burden of chronic kidney disease (CKD) continues to increase, the use of the most cost-effective modality of KRT is imperative in all economies in the world. Despite that, there are some regional differences in the incidence and prevalence of the most commonly used modalities of KRT worldwide.

The 2018 International Society of Nephrology Global Kidney Health Atlas (ISN-GKHA) reported that the median global prevalence of peritoneal dialysis (PD) was 38.1 per million population (pmp), accounting for 11% of all patients receiving dialysis and 9% of all patients on KRT in the world. However, the prevalence of PD varied from 0.1 pmp in Egypt to 531 pmp in Hong Kong. More than half of all patients receiving PD were concentrated in four countries (China, USA, Mexico, and Thailand).

The reasons for global differences in the utilization of PD are complex and related to variable factors:

- Availability of PD: PD was not available in 30 countries, 20 of them were located in Africa.
- Patient factors: visual acuity, mobility, cognitive ability, family support, financial status.
- Facility factors: physician bias and experience, physician availability, surgeon availability, infrastructure support for urgent-start PD, PD, and HD training processes.
- Health care system factors: public vs. private models, financial incentives, dialysis policy.
- Industry factors: local fluid manufacture, solution costs.

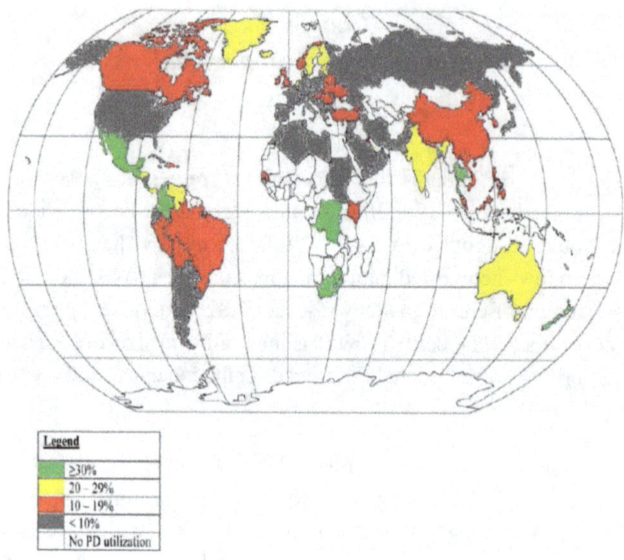

**Figure 1.** Prevalence of utilization of PD across the globe in the year 2015. (Abraham G et al. A review of acute and chronic peritoneal dialysis in developing countries. Clin Kidney J. 2015 Jun;8(3):310-307.)

Current estimates suggest that more than 272,000 patients receive PD worldwide (approximately 11% of the global dialysis population) with an annual global growth rate of PD utilization of 8%, which is higher than that of hemodialysis (6–7%). Mexico, the United States, and China had the absolute largest number of patients receiving PD in the world. In four countries, Hong Kong, El Salvador, Mexico, and Guatemala, the majority of dialysis patients were treated with PD. Hong Kong had the highest prevalence of PD per million population, followed by Mexico and El Salvador (Figure 1).

Despite some differences in the utilization of PD between developing and developed countries, a simple linear correlation between the wealth of the country and the percentage of PD use could not be established. A recent international survey study based on data collected from 156 countries (85% of the global population) showed that PD use was 60-fold lower in low-income countries (LICs) (0.9 pmp, 95% CI 0.7–1.5) than in high-income countries (HICs) (53.0 pmp, 95% CI 40.6–89.8 pmp). However, further country-by-country analysis showed that among HICs, the proportion of patients receiving PD ranged from a high of 25% in Canada and Australia, to a low of

3% in Japan. Similarly, whereas most LICs have <10% utilization of PD, three countries in this income category (Mexico, Guatemala, and Thailand) used PD in 28%–59% of their patients receiving dialysis. PD was not available in 30 of the 156 (19%) countries, predominately in Africa (20/41) and LICs (15/22). In 69% of the countries, PD was the initial dialysis modality for less than 10% of patients with newly diagnosed kidney failure. Patients receiving PD need to pay from 1% to 25% of the treatment costs, with the highest copayments in South Asia and LICs.

There was a substantial variation in the type of PD used across countries. The number of PD patients treated with automated peritoneal dialysis (APD) was significantly lower in developing countries compared with developed countries. APD was used in 15.8% of PD patients in developing countries and 42.4% of the patients in developed countries. Over the past two decades, there has been an increase in the use of APD in both developing and developed countries.

The dialysis policy appeared to be the greatest determinant of the proportion of patients treated with PD. The greater cost-effectiveness of PD compared to HD (in the most countries) has stimulated some countries to implement policies and financial incentives that favor the use of PD. PD-favored policies regarding their background might be grouped as follows:

- PD-First: PD is used as the first treatment modality for all appropriate KF patients. Switching to hemodialysis is only permitted if peritoneal dialysis fails.
- PD-Favored: In these countries, patient, provider, and payer incentives favored the use of PD as the treatment modality.
- Home Dialysis-First policies (including PD and home HD)

The review of literature and local government policies showed that countries like Hong Kong and Thailand have PD-First policies. Canada, China, Guatemala, India, Mexico, Spain, Taiwan, and the United States have PD-Favored policies. Australia, Finland, and New Zealand were identified as having Home Dialysis-First policies. These policies are important for developing countries where there is a high rate of KF patients, but resources and access to in-center hemodialysis are limited. For example, in Mexico, this policy has been extremely successful, with 59% of patients on KRT using PD, which led to substantial healthcare savings. In 2007, Thailand introduced the PD–first policy after which there was an exponential growth in the number of Thai patients with PD, from 1198 to 26,450 patients.

Analyzes showed that the prevalence of peritoneal dialysis is inversely correlated with the increasing number of hemodialysis units near patients' homes. In many countries, the development of HD units led to a decrease in the utilization of PD. For example, in Israel, peritoneal dialysis use decreased from 34% in 1990 to 7% in 2015 as a consequence of the increasing number of HD units that offered accessibility and convenience for the patients. Moreover, the authors concluded that the growing elderly dialysis population in HICs enjoyed the social aspects of in-center hemodialysis and regular medical monitoring in the centers. Similarly, in Korea, as the number of HD units doubled between 2006 and 2018, the proportion of patients that received peritoneal dialysis decreased from 22% to 7% during the same period.

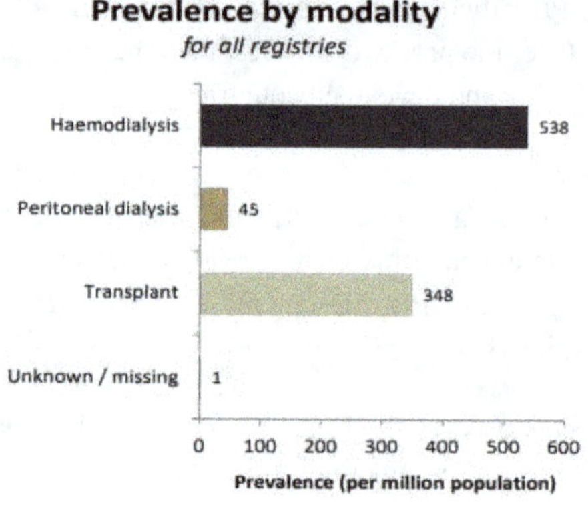


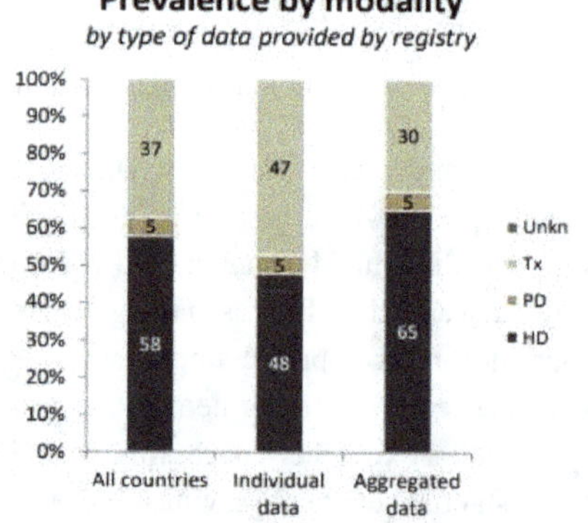


**Figure 2.** Prevalence of modality of RRT in European countries according to ERA/EDTA Annual Report for the year 2020 in which data from 52 national or regional renal registries in 34 countries.

There are large disparities in PD availability, accessibility, affordability, and delivery among countries in the world. The dialysis policy in a country appeared to be the greatest determinant of the proportion of patients treated with PD. The prevalence of the modality of KRT in European countries including North Macedonia according to the ERA/EDTA Annual Report is given in Figure 2 and Table 1 respectively.

**Table 1.** The trend of KRT in the last 6 years in North Macedonia

| Years | Total | Etiology of Kidney Disease | | | | | | | | Type of KRT | | |
|---|---|---|---|---|---|---|---|---|---|---|---|---|
| | | GN | PN | PKD | DM | HTA | RV | Mis | Unk | HD | PD | Tx |
| 2020 | 1762 | 263 | 124 | 166 | 312 | 473 | 6 | 171 | 247 | 1514 | 17 | 231 |
| 2019 | 1853 | 284 | 141 | 176 | 329 | 483 | 19 | 183 | 238 | 1608 | 17 | 228 |
| 2018 | 1756 | 296 | 168 | 157 | 304 | 454 | 3 | 144 | 230 | 1488 | 19 | 249 |
| 2017 | 1761 | 297 | 160 | 166 | 200 | 446 | 2 | 142 | 248 | 1521 | 22 | 218 |
| 2016 | 1665 | 290 | 152 | 163 | 273 | 414 | 3 | 155 | 215 | 1433 | 25 | 207 |
| 2015 | 1598 | 253 | 125 | 165 | 245 | 389 | 2 | 216 | 202 | 1353 | 32 | 213 |

*GN - glomerulonephritis; PN - pyelonephritis; PKD - polycystic kidney disease; HTA - hypertension, RV - renovascular disease; Mis – Miscellaneous; Unk- Unknown; HD - hemodialysis; PD - peritoneal dialysis, Tx - transplantation. (Gjorgjievski N, Karanfilovski V. Global Dialysis Perspective: North Macedonia. Kidney360. 2023 Apr 1;4(4):e525-e529.)

**References**

1. Liyanage T, Ninomiya T, Jha V. Worldwide access to treatment for end-stage kidney disease: a systematic review. Lancet. 2015;385:1975–1982.
2. Li PK, Chow KM, Van de Luijtgaarden MW, Johnson DW, Jager KJ, Mehrotra R et al. Changes in the worldwide epidemiology of peritoneal dialysis. Nat Rev Nephrol. 2017 Feb;13(2):90-103.
3. Bello AK, Okpechi IG, Osman MA, Cho Y, Cullis B, Htay H, et al. Epidemiology of peritoneal dialysis outcomes. Nat Rev Nephrol. 2022 Dec;18(12):779-793.
4. Cho Y, Bello AK, Levin A, Lunney M, Osman MA, Ye F et al. Peritoneal Dialysis Use and Practice Patterns: An International Survey Study. Am J Kidney Dis. 2021 Mar;77(3):315-325.
5. Jain AK, Blake P, Cordy P, Garg AX. Global trends in rates of peritoneal dialysis. J Am Soc Nephrol. 2012 Mar;23(3):533-544.
6. Timmy F.L, Jennifer E, Allon M. Dialysis Care around the World: A Global Perspectives Series. Kidney360. 2021 April; 2(4):604-607.
7. Megan E A, Rianne B, Abd El Hafeez S, Trujillo-Alemán S, Federico A, Anders Å et al. The ERA Registry Annual Report 2020: a summary, Clinical Kid J. 2023 Aug;16(8):1330–1354.
8. Pecoits-Filho R, Okpechi IG, Donner JA, Harris DCH, Aljubori HM, Bello AK et al. Capturing and monitoring global differences in untreated and treated end-stage kidney disease, kidney replacement therapy modality, and outcomes. Kidney Int Suppl. 2020 Mar;10(1):e3-e9.
9. Liu FX, Gao X, Inglese G, Chuengsaman P, Pecoits-Filho R, Yu A. A Global Overview of the Impact of Peritoneal Dialysis First or Favored Policies: An Opinion. Perit Dial Int. 2015 Jul-Aug;35(4):406-420.
10. Gjorgjievski N, Karanfilovski V. Global Dialysis Perspective: North Macedonia. Kidney360. 2023 Apr 1;4(4):e525-e529.

*Chapter 3*
*Principles of peritoneal dialysis*

## 3.1.  The peritoneal membrane

The peritoneal membrane is the dialyzing surface in the peritoneal dialysis (PD). The peritoneum is a serosal membrane that lines the peritoneal cavity. The peritoneum approximates body surface area in size and typically ranges from 1 to 2 $m^2$ in an adult. Anatomically, it is composed of two layers: the visceral peritoneum, which covers the abdominal organs and accounts for 80% of the total surface area, and the parietal peritoneum, which lines the undersurface of the diaphragm and the interior surface of the anterior abdominal wall. The peritoneal membrane is a semi-permeable, bi-directional, highly vascularized structure. Histologically, the peritoneum consists of the superficial layer of mesothelial cells and a deep layer of gel-like interstitial tissue composed of fibroblasts, macrophages, lymphatic and blood vessels (Figure 1).

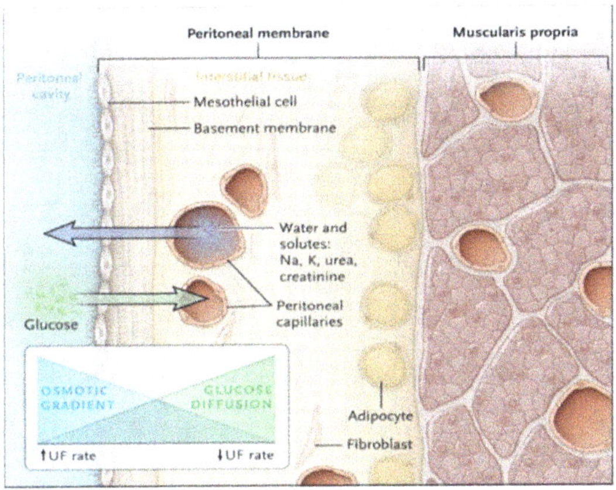


**Figure 1.** Anatomy and basic physiological processes during PD (Isaac Teitelbaum. Peritoneal Dialysis. N Engl J Med 2021; 385:1786-1795)

It is believed that the endothelium, which builds the wall of the mentioned capillaries, is the main barrier for the transport of water and substances during PD. The mesothelial cells are covered by microvilli that provide greater peritoneal surface area (size of $1.5 - 2$ $m^2$). The effective surface area necessary to achieve PD depends on the surface area of the peritoneal membrane and its vascularity.

## 3.2. Physiology of Peritoneal Dialysis

There is an exchange of fluid and solutes across the semipermeable peritoneal membrane between the blood in peritoneal capillaries and the dialysis solution installed into the peritoneal cavity (Figure 1). The process of filling and draining the peritoneal cavity with dialysate is called an exchange. The length of time the dialysate remains in the peritoneal cavity is called the dwell time. During the dwell of dialysate, the waste products (urea, creatinine) move from the blood in peritoneal capillaries into the dialysate, whereas glucose and lactate move from the dialysate into the blood in peritoneal capillaries (bi-directional movement), Figure 1. The standard PD dialysis fluid contains sodium, chloride, calcium, magnesium, dextrose (D-glucose) as an osmolyte, and lactate as a buffer.

**Table 1.** Composition of standard peritoneal dialysis fluid

| Osmotic agents* | | |
|---|---|---|
| Glucose | (g/dl) | 1.5, 2.5 or 4,25 |
| Amino acids | (g/dL) | 1.1 |
| Icodextrin | (g/dL) | 7.5 |
| **Buffer**** | | |
| Lactate | (mEq/l) | 36.5 – 40 |
| Bicarbonate | (mEq/l) | 0-34 |
| **Electrolytes** | | |
| Sodium | (mEq/l) | 132 – 133 |
| Potassium | (mEq/l) | 0 – 2 |
| Calcium | (mEq/l) | 2.5-3.5 |
| Magnesium | (mEq/l) | 0.5 |
| Chloride | (mEq/l) | 95 – 101 |
| pH | | 5.2 – 7.4 |
| Osmolality | mOsmol/L | 282 – 485 |

* Current osmotic agents include glucose, amino acids, or icodextrin.
** Either bicarbonate or lactate serves as a buffer, in a total concentration not exceeding 40 mEq/l.
(Vardhan A., Hutchinson J.A. Peritoneal dialysis. In: Scott J. Gilbert and Daniel E. Weiner. Primer of kidney diseases. Elsevier. 2014. 6th edition, pp 523.)

Peritoneal dialysis involves three transport mechanisms: diffusion, ultrafiltration, and convection through the highly vascularized peritoneal membrane. The removal of solutes from blood to dialysis fluid through the peritoneal membrane is achieved by diffusion (solute movement down a concentration gradient) and convection (solute movement that accompanies ultrafiltration). The diffusion of solutes is the fastest in the first hour after installation of dialysis fluid and becomes slower as the gradients decline over time. By the 4th hour, more than 90% of urea and more than 65% of creatinine is equilibrated in the majority of the patients.

Ultrafiltration during PD is achieved by dextrose (D-glucose), the main osmotic agent in the dialysis fluid with osmotic power, simple metabolism, and safety. There are dialysis fluids with different concentrations of glucose. The glucose-based dialysate fluids are hyperosmolar to plasma. The different concentrations of glucose determine the gradient for ultrafiltration. The higher concentrations of glucose drive more water movement from the blood into the peritoneal cavity during a dwell. There is also transperitoneal absorption of the glucose from dialysate in the blood during the dwelling (Figure 1). Consequently, there is a decrease in the concentration of glucose in the dialysate with a decrease in the osmotic gradient and ultrafiltration potential of the dialysate.

### 3.3.  The three-pore model of peritoneal dialysis

In the three-pore model, the peritoneal transport of solutes and fluid depends on the relative number of three types of pores with variable sizes in capillary endothelium (Figure 2):

- **Large pores** (radius of  20 - 40 nm) are gaps between venular endothelial cells and represent only 0.5% of total number of pores. These pores are involved in the transport of macromolecules, small molecules, and partly in ultrafiltration which is achieved by convection of plasma from blood to the peritoneal cavity.
- **Small pores** (radius of 4 - 6 nm) correspond to the clefts or gaps located between endothelial cells and account for ~95% of all pores. The transport of small molecules (urea, creatinine, electrolytes) and to a lesser extent water is realized through this type of pores.
- **Ultrasmall pores** (radius of < 0.8 nm) correspond to aquaporin channels (AQP-1) in the endothelial cell membrane. They account only for 1–2% of all pores, but ~50% of the total UF occurs through these pores.

The rate of removal of solutes through the peritoneal membrane depends on the concentration gradient and the degree of vascularization of the membrane. In patients with poorer peritoneal vascularization, the removal of solutes from blood into dialysate fluid is slow but the ultrafiltration rate is relatively good because glucose absorption from dialysate fluid to blood is also low. Conversely, in patients with greater vascularization of the peritoneal membrane, the removal of solutes from blood in the dialysate fluid is fast, but the ultrafiltration is poor because of the fast absorption of glucose from the dialysate into the blood. With the use of non-glucose-based dialysis fluid with icodextrin as an osmotic agent that does not diffuse through the peritoneal membrane, the ultrafiltration process could be maintained for up to 13 to 16 hours.

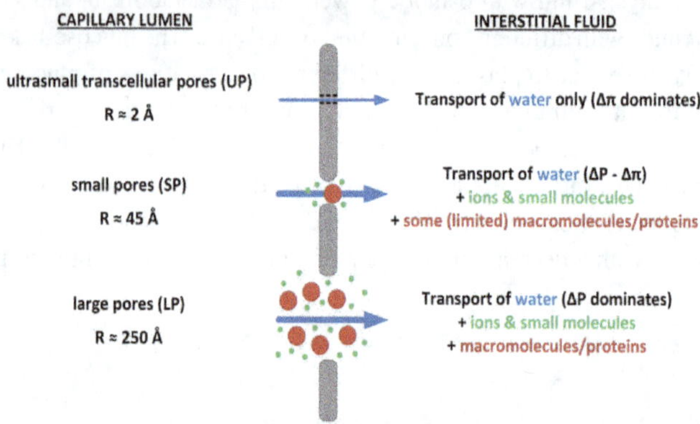


**Figure 2.** The three-pore model of the transcapillary transport of water, small solutes, and macromolecules. ΔP – differences in hydrostatic pressure difference between capillary blood and interstitial fluid; Δπ – differences in osmotic pressure difference between plasma and interstitial fluid. (Pstras, Leszek & Waniewski, Jacek & Lindholm, Bengt. (2020). Transcapillary transport of water, small solutes, and proteins during hemodialysis.)

The rate of removal of solutes through the peritoneal membrane also depends on molecular weight, protein-binding, and net charge of the solutes. The serum proteins (albumin) with high molecular weight are transported slowly through the peritoneal membrane. The protein loss with PD is approximately 6–8 g per day and could be significantly increased during episodes of peritonitis. Dialysis clearances of the middle molecule beta-microglobulin and the protein-bound solute p-cresol are less effective than the removal of small molecules and usually require longer dwell time. The peritoneal membrane has a net negative charge and negatively charged solutes like phosphates move through it less effectively.

More recent studies show that certain genetic polymorphisms could affect the rate of water and solute transport across the peritoneal membrane. Morelle J et al. demonstrated that a single nucleotide polymorphism (rs2075574) of the aquaporin channel-1 gene was associated with peritoneal ultrafiltration. Other authors showed increased expression of SGLT-2 transporters in patients with long-term PD, especially in those who developed encapsulating peritoneal sclerosis. It is assumed that the use of SGLT-2 inhibitors could have a potential benefit on the preservation of the peritoneal membrane. Epigenetic modifications such as DNA methylation and histone modification could influence the development of peritoneal fibrosis associated with poor ultrafiltration and technique failure.

## 3.4.  Peritoneal membrane preservation

High concentrations of glucose and glucose degradation products (GDPs) in standard dialysate fluid cause increased production of inflammatory cytokines that aggravate chronic inflammation and result in peritoneal fibrosis, damage of the peritoneal membrane, and technique failure. Many different cytokines and growth factors lead to the epithelial-to-mesenchymal transition of mesothelial cells, fibrosis, and neoangiogenesis with irreversible changes of the peritoneal membrane (Figure 3).

Many strategies have been proposed to prevent the remodeling of the peritoneal membrane that occur during the long-term PD treatment:

- **Use of biocompatible PD solutions:** with neutral pH and low glucose degradation products.
- **Low-glucose PD regimens – icodextrin and amino acid:** Repeated exposure of the peritoneal membrane to high concentrations of glucose results in sclerosis of the peritoneum. Low-glucose PD regimen including solutions with icodextrin and amino acids as osmotic agents could be associated with better preservation of the peritoneal membrane.
- **Peritoneal resting:** temporal transfer to hemodialysis.
- **Renin-Angiotensin-Aldosterone System blockade agents:** blockage of RAAS decreases the local production of cytokines and formation of fibrosis.
- **Heparin and other glycosaminoglycans:** Fibrin was a matrix for the initiation of peritoneal fibrotic processes. Heparin shows immunomodulatory effects, effects on the extracellular matrix, and antiangiogenic, anti-inflammatory, antiproliferative, and anti-fibrotic properties.

- **Agents targeting epithelial-to-mesenchymal transition of mesothelial cells:** agents blocking TGF-β1 and other cytokines, Tamoxifen, Celecoxib (inhibitor of COX-2), Rosiglitazone (reduced effects of GDPs in the formation of AGEs).
- **Alternative osmotic agents:** experimental studies with use of L-carnitine and taurine show promising results.

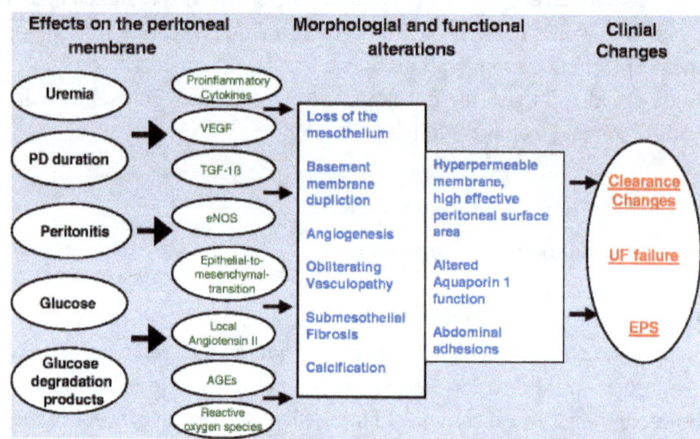



**Figure 3**. Morphological and functional changes of peritoneal membrane and associated clinical consequences in long-term PD. (AGEs – advanced glycosylation end products; VEGF – vascular endothelial growth factor; eNOS - endothelial nitric oxide synthase, TGF-1β-transforming growth factor-β, UF-ultrafiltration, EPS- encapsulating peritoneal sclerosis). (Fusshoeller, A. Histomorphological and functional changes of the peritoneal membrane during long-term peritoneal dialysis. Pediatr Nephrol. 2008;(23):19–25)

**References**

1. Farooqi S, Baqir D, Naqvi S, Gauhar Dr. Stability study of antibiotic (cefotaxime) in peritoneal dialysis solution with validation of analyzing method. International Journal of Pharmacy and Pharmaceutical Sciences. 2013;(5):930-934.
2. Morelle J, Marechal C, Yu Z, Debaix H, Corre T, Lambie M et al. AQP1 Promoter Variant, Water Transport, and Outcomes in Peritoneal Dialysis. N. Engl. J. Med. 2021;385:1570–1580.
3. Isaac Teitelbaum. Peritoneal Dialysis. N Engl J Med 2021; 385:1786-1795.
4. Chen C.H., Teitelbaum I. Physiology of Peritoneal Dialysis. In: Rastogi A., Lerma E.V., Bargman J.M., editors. Applied Peritoneal Dialysis: Improving Patient Outcomes. Springer International Publishing; Cham, Switzerland: 2021. pp. 11–23.
5. Kunin M, Beckerman P. The Peritoneal Membrane Potential Mediator of Fibrosis and Inflammation among Heart Failure Patients on Peritoneal Dialysis. Membranes (Basel). 2022 Mar 11;12(3):318.
6. Devuyst O, Goffin E. Water and solute transport in peritoneal dialysis: models and clinical applications, Nephrology Dialysis Transplantation. 2008 July.23(7):2120–2123.
7. Rippe B. A three-pore model of peritoneal transport. Perit Dial Int. 1993;13(2):S35-38.
8. Rippe B, Simonsen O, Stelin G. Clinical implications of a three-pore model of peritoneal transport. Adv Perit Dial. 1991;7:3-9.
9. Fusshoeller, A. Histomorphological and functional changes of the peritoneal membrane during long-term peritoneal dialysis. Pediatr Nephrol. 2008; 23:19–25.
10. Bajo, M. A, del Peso, G, Teitelbaum, I. Peritoneal Membrane Preservation. Seminars in Nephrology. 2017;37(1):77–92.

*Chapter 4*
*Catheters for peritoneal dialysis*

A well-placed and functioning peritoneal dialysis (PD) catheter is essential for the success of peritoneal dialysis. PD catheter is an access for performing peritoneal dialysis, like vascular access for hemodialysis. It travels through the patient's abdominal wall and cavity and presents a tool through which an exchange of peritoneal dialysis solutions is achieved. Complications related to the PD catheter are associated with the morbidity and mortality of PD patients and are major causes of PD failure. In the Netherlands Cooperative Study on the Adequacy of Dialysis (NECOSAD), abdominal and catheter complications accounted for 40% of transfers from PD to HD during the first 3 months of PD initiation, with a decrease to 25% after 2 years of PD treatment. Peritoneal access failure was the reason for approximately 20–35% of PD technical failures (dropouts from PD to HD). The knowledge of best practices in PD-catheter placement and care could optimize these complications and provide better PD outcomes.

## 4.1 History of peritoneal access development

- **Late 1940s**: Ferris and Odel designed a soft, polyvinyl intraperitoneal tube with metal weights to keep the catheter tip in the pelvic gutter where the conditions for drain are the best.
- **In the 1950's:** polyethylene and nylon catheters became commercially available. PD was used for the treatment of acute renal failure.
- **In the 1960's:** silicon rubber was discovered which is less irritating to the peritoneal membrane. Polyester velour and polyester cuff were developed which provided restricted catheter movement and created a closed tunnel between the integument and the peritoneal cavity.
- **In 1968:** Tenckhoff and Schechter combined the two previously mentioned achievements and developed a silicone rubber catheter with a polyester cuff for treatment of acute kidney failure and two cuffs for treatment of chronic kidney failure. This was a technological revolution in access for PD.
- Even today, **Tenckhoff catheters** with some modifications continue to be widely used for PD access.

- **Swan-neck catheters** with an inverted U-shaped arc and a downward exit were developed to reduce the risk of exit-site infections, tip migration, and protrusion of the subcutaneous cuff.

## 4.2. Characteristics of an ideal PD catheter

PD catheter should provide:

- Optimal inflow and outflow of dialysate fluids
- Kink resistance without displacement and fluid leakage
- Biocompatibility without causing inflammation, sclerosis, and adhesions of the peritoneal membrane
- Optimal protection against microorganisms, preventing exit-site infection and peritonitis
- Easy to implant and remove
- Low cost

## 4.3. Types of PD catheters

The most widely used PD catheters have three segments:

- **External segment**: the part that is outside the body and is visible (Figure 3)
- **Tunneled segment:** the part of the catheter that goes through the abdominal wall
- **Intra-peritoneal segment:** the part of the catheter which is placed in the peritoneal cavity

Several types of PD catheters are available for use: catheters with different intraperitoneal parts (straight or coiled), different subcutaneous segments (prefabricated bend (swan neck) or straight (Tenckhoff)), and with number of cuffs on the catheters (single or double cuff). The intra-peritoneal part of the catheter consists of a flexible silicone tube with an open-end port and several side holes for drainage and absorption of the dialysate. The tunneled segment of the PD catheter has either one or two Dacron cuffs.

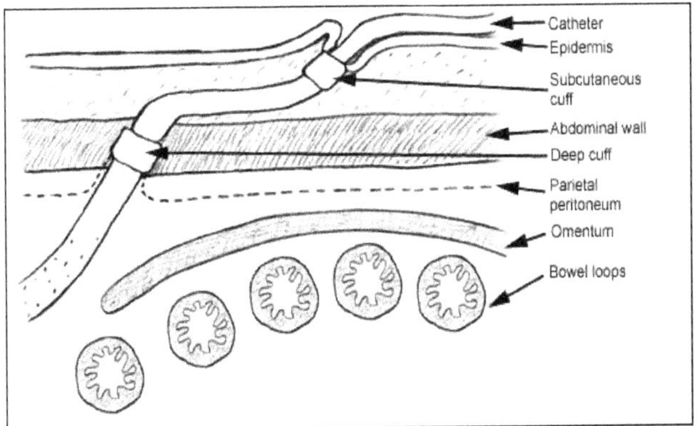



**Figure 1.** Schematic of a straight-tip Tenckhoff peritoneal catheter and its relationship to adjacent anatomic structures. (Crabtree, J. H., & Chow, K.-M. Peritoneal Dialysis Catheter Insertion. Seminars in Nephrology. 2017. 37(1): 17–29.)

Most catheters have a double cuff: the deep cuff which is implanted in the preperitoneal space (muscle) and holds the catheter in place and the subcutaneous cuff which is implanted in the subcutaneous tissue and serves as a barrier to infection (Figure 1, Figure 2).

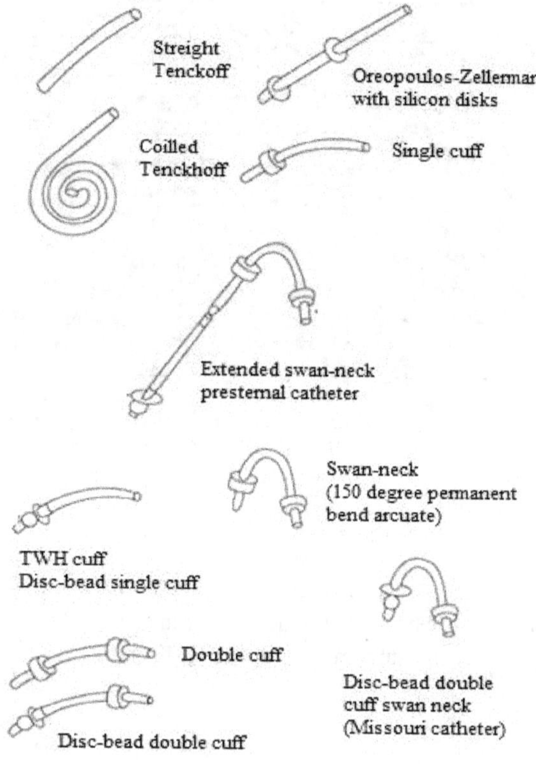


**Figure 2.** The most commonly used types of peritoneal catheters

## 4.4. Selection of PD catheter

There is no preferred type of PD catheter. In the literature, there was no clear evidence of whether one specific type of catheter was superior regarding PD outcomes. The largest available meta-analysis performed by Hagen M.S. et al. included three comparisons: straight vs. coiled catheters, straight vs. swan neck, and single vs. double cuff catheters in terms of catheter survival, drainage dysfunction, migration, leakage, exit-site infections, peritonitis, and catheter removal.

- **Intra-peritoneal segment of PD catheter: coiled vs. straight**

Based on data from 454 patients, there was no statistically significant difference between the group with coiled and the group with straight catheters in the rate of exit-site infection, the incidence of peritonitis episodes, the incidence of migration, leakage, and catheter removal. The survival of the catheters at 1 year post insertion was not significantly different between the groups, but the survival at 2 years post insertion was significantly different in favor of straight catheters.

- **Subcutaneous segment of PD catheter: straight vs. swan neck**

There was no difference in the incidence of exit-site infections, risk of developing peritonitis, migration, leakage, removal and catheter dysfunction between patients with straight or swan neck subcutaneous segments.

- The tunneled segment of the PD catheter with the **number of cuffs: single cuff vs. double cuff**

There was no significant difference in the incidence of catheter survival, episodes of peritonitis, and exit-site infections between catheters with single or double cuffs.

The choice of the best catheter type for PD is a balance between the pelvic location of the catheter tip and the exit site which should be easily accessible for proper care. The patient's belt line, obesity, skin creases, and folds, presence of scars, chronic skin conditions, incontinence, physical limitations, bathing habits, and occupation should be also taken into consideration.

### 4.4.1. Determination of catheter insertion site

The patient is in the supine position. For a coiled-tip catheter, the upper border of the catheter coil should be aligned with the upper border of the pubic symphysis. The upper border of the deep cuff indicates the location of the insertion incision (Figure 3). Paramedian location (2-4 cm below or above and left of the umbilicus) is preferred with a deep cuff tunneled into the rectus muscle that prevents displacement of the catheter and leakage. In this way, the catheter-associated discomfort, early termination of dialysate outflow from compression-obstruction, and severe end-of-drain pain are reduced to a minimum. The insert location for straight-tip catheters is more flexible, but the periumbilical location is also the most commonly used.

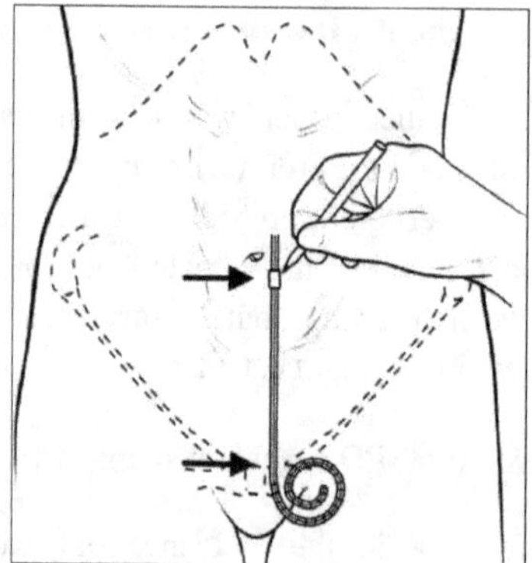

**Figure 3.** Scheme of the coiled-tip catheter insertion site and deep cuff location to achieve proper pelvic position of the catheter tip. (Peppelenbosch et al. Peritoneal dialysis catheter placement technique and complications. NDT Plus 1. 2008: iv23 - iv28.)

## 4.4.2. Determination of tunnel configuration and exit site location

In swan-neck bend catheter, the subcutaneous tunnel path and exit site location follows the configuration of the tube, and the skin exit site is 2 to 3 cm beyond the superficial cuff. Catheters with a straight intercuff segment should form a gentle arc in the subcutaneous tissues to produce more laterally directed exit site. Upwardly directed exit sites should be avoided for prevention of bacterial collection. For patients with severe obesity and multiple abdominal skin folds, an upper abdominal exit site or extended catheter with a presternal exit site might be considered.

## 4.5. Techniques for PD catheter placement

Peritoneal dialysis catheters might be placed into abdominal cavity via a percutaneous, a laparoscopic, or an open surgical technique.

- **Open surgical technique**

During this procedure, the patient is in a supine position and general anesthesiaa is used. Vertical, 2-3 cm long, infra umbilical midleline incision is made with subsequent dissection of the rectus abdominal muscle. The posterior sheath of the muscle is incised and the abdominal cavity is opened after dissecting the peritoneum.

The patient is placed in a Trendelenburg position, and the catheter is placed into the peritoneal cavity by using a stylet. The deep cuff is positioned in the preperitoneal space, and the peritoneum and posterior and anterior rectus sheaths are closed with absorbable sutures. A tunnel is created to the exit site, usually lateral and caudal to the entrance site. The subcutaneous cuff is placed 2 cm from the exit site. The procedure is completed by testing the catheter with inflow of 100 ml sterile saline. The saline is then drained and inspected to ensure no intraperitoneal bleeding or fecal contamination.

- **Laparoscopic technique**

The laparoscopic technique is minimally invasive and provides an opportunity to perform partial omentectomy or lysis of adhesions if needed during the catheter placement. Pneumoperitoneum is created with insufflation of $CO_2$ by using a 5 mm trocar inserted into the abdomen via a small subumbilical incision or by using the Veres needle technique. Then the patient is placed in the Trendelenburg position and a diagnostic laparoscopy is performed. At the planned exit-site position (paraumbilical region) an additional 5-mm trocar is placed in preperitoneal space (not in peritoneal cavity). A double-cuffed curled tip peritoneal dialysis catheter is placed into the pouch of Douglas through the subumbilical port by using a stylet. The distal cuff is positioned between the rectus sheaths. The paraumbilical trocar is removed, and the catheter is placed through the created subcutaneous tunnel toward the second trocar. The proximal, subcutaneous cuff is positioned within the tunnel 2-3 cm from the exit-site. The catheter is tested, and the abdomen is desufflated. The trocar is removed, and the rectus sheaths are closed carefully with resorbable sutures.

- **Percutaneous technique**

The percutaneous placement of PD catheter is done by using the modified Seldinger technique, usually under local anesthesia and often at the bedside. An 18-gauge introduction needle and a guide wire are placed into the abdomen in the paramedian location. The abdomen is filled with 500 ml saline. The needle is removed, and a dilator and a peel-away sheath are advanced over the wire into the abdominal cavity. Serial dilatation is performed. The guidewire and dilator are removed. To facilitate insertion, the PD catheter is straightened and stiffened by insertion of an internal stylet and placed through the sheath in the pelvis. The peel-away sheath and stylet are removed and the catheter position is checked. The deep cuff is advanced to the level of the muscle fascia. With a tunneling tool, a subcutaneous tunnel to the designated skin exit site is created in which the proximal, subcutaneous cuff is positioned. The entrance site is closed.

A review of the outcomes of percutaneous versus open surgical placement of PD catheters demonstrates similar results regarding the risk of peritonitis, catheter removal or replacement, technical failure, and all-cause mortality. However, a recent meta-analysis demonstrated that the percutaneous method performed better with fewer overall mechanical complications and less malposition than open surgery. The leakage risk was higher in the blind percutaneous group, while the guided percutaneous placement group showed similar outcomes to the surgical method groups. Percutaneous methods also had a lower infection risk, which needs further evidence to be confirmed. Moreover, another study showed that the incision size ($2.6 \pm 0.7$ vs $7.3 \pm 0.6$ cm) and the length of hospital stay ($11.9 \pm 5.9$ vs $17.3 \pm 6.8$ d) were considerably less in the percutaneously placed group compared to the surgically placed group. Percutaneous PD-catheter placement allows a rapid initiation of CAPD, and avoids the necessity for operating room time, and the requirement for a peritoneal incision. It has a high technical success rate and could be performed on an outpatient basis or in patients who cannot tolerate general anesthesia.

Peppelenbosch A. et al. recommended using of laparoscopic technique in patients with previous abdominal surgery because it provides an opportunity for additional adhesiolysis and removal of omental wrapping or fibrin clotting from the catheter.

## 4.6. Complications of PD catheter placement

### 4.6.1. Early complications (occurred in first 30 days after placement)

- **Bowel or urinary bladder perforation** (in less than 1% of the patients).
- **Bleeding** (relatively common complication but severe bleeding is encountered in only 1% to 5% of procedures). Pericannular bleeding close to the exit site is the most common form and is managed with manual pressure, additional suturing, and local administration of epinephrine or desmopressin acetate. Rectus sheath hematoma also has been observed after PD catheter insertion.
- **Mechanical flow dysfunction:** kinking, omental wrapping, ensnaring by adhesions, migration of the catheter tip, and catheter displacement. The management includes irrigation with saline or urokinase, laparoscopy with omentectomy, adhesiolysis, and repositioning.
- **Leakage of dialysate:** the most common complication, with a reported frequency as high as 12.8%. Catheter rest without dialysate instillation for several weeks could most likely solve this complication.

*4.6.2. Late complications (occurred  30 days after placement)*

The late complications related to PD catheter are exit-site infection, tunnel infection, cuff protrusion, outflow failure, and dialysate leaks or hernias. These complications are presented in the respective chapters.


## 4.7. Care for PD catheter

After insertion, PD catheters should undergo irrigation with 1000 ml peritoneal dialysate solution within 3 days to wash out the blood and fibrinous debris. The irrigation should be repeated until clear effluent is achieved. Adding heparin in dialysate solution might help prevent fibrin and blood coagulum from plugging into the catheter. It was widely adopted that PD catheter insertion should be performed at least 2 weeks before starting with PD treatment. It is believed that during this "break-in" period the wounds were healing and the mechanical complications (mostly leakage) were less common compared to an early or urgent start of PD. These findings were based mainly on expert opinions, and the conclusions of the studies were uncertain. A recent case series of 657 PD patients showed that patients with a break-in period of 7 days or fewer experienced a slightly higher risk of catheter dysfunction compared to those with a break-in period of more than 2 weeks (8.4% vs. 1.7%). However, there was no major effect on technique survival between both groups. The patients might perform only mild physical activities for 4 to 6 weeks after PD placement. The exit site should be daily clean by nonirritating, antiseptic agents followed by aplication of antibiotic ointment (mupirocin, gentamicin), and sterile dressings over the exit site. Swimming was not advised in the first 3-4 weeks.


## 4.8. PD catheter inserted by a nephrologist

PD catheter is inserted into the abdominal cavity either by a surgeon, interventional radiologist or nephrologist. Nephrologists used less invasive peritoneoscopic or percutaneous techniques for insertion. Beside the above mentioned advantages of using non-surgical methodes, the potential advantages of PD catheters placed by nephrologists included better continuity of care, reduced waiting times, and the creation of a committed nephrology team with particular interest in PD.

**References**

1. Crabtree JH, Chow KM. Peritoneal Dialysis Catheter Insertion. Semin Nephrol. 2017 Jan;37(1):17-29.
2. Twardowski ZJ. History of peritoneal access development. Int J Artif Organs. 2006 Jan;29(1):2-40.
3. Twardowski ZJ. Peritoneal access: the past, present, and the future. Contrib Nephrol. 2006;150:195-201.
4. Linxi Huang, Cheng Xue, Sixiu Chen, Shoulian Zhou, Bo Yang, Mengna Ruan, et al. Comparison of Outcomes between Percutaneous and Surgical Placement of Peritoneal Dialysis Catheters in Uremic Patients: A Meta-Analysis. Blood Purif. April 2022; 51(4):328–344.
5. Gallieni M, Giordano A, Pinerolo C, Cariati M. Type of peritoneal dialysis catheter and outcomes. J Vasc Access. 2015;16(9):S68-72.
6. Pandya YK, Wagner JK, Yuo T, Eslami M, Singh MJ, Hager ES. Outcomes of peritoneal dialysis catheter configurations and pelvic fixation. Surg Open Sci. 2019 May 18;1(1):34-37.
7. Peppelenbosch A, van Kuijk WH, Bouvy ND, van der Sande FM, Tordoir JH. Peritoneal dialysis catheter placement technique and complications. NDT Plus. 2008 Oct;1(4):iv23-iv28.
8. Sander M. Hagen, Jeffrey A. Lafranca, Jan N.M. Ijzermans, Frank J.M.F. Dor. A systematic review and meta-analysis of the influence of peritoneal dialysis catheter type on complication rate and catheter survival. Kidney International. 2014; 85(4):920-932.
9. Kache SA, Sale D, Makama JG. Techniques for Peritoneal Dialysis Catheter Placement. Evolving Strategies in Peritoneal Dialysis. InTech; 2018.
10. Sampathkumar K, Mahaldar AR, Sooraj YS, Ramkrishnan M, Ajeshkumar, Ravichandran R. Percutaneous CAPD catheter insertion by a nephrologist versus surgical placement: A comparative study. Indian J Nephrol. 2008 Jan;18(1):5-8.

*Chapter 5*
*Techniques of peritoneal dialysis*

## 5.1 Continuous Ambulatory Peritoneal Dialysis (CAPD)

CAPD is a commonly used PD technique that involves the manual instillation of dialysis fluid (up to 3 L) into the peritoneal cavity through a pre-implanted PD catheter. Peritoneal dialysis fluid is installed by gravity and after a dwell time of several hours is drained in an empty bag. The CAPD treatment is presented with two to four short-dwell exchanges during the day and one long dwell overnight. The prescription of the type of dialysis fluid, the volume, the dwell time, and the number of exchanges is individual for every patient, depending on the body surface of the patient, the peritoneal membrane transport type, and the residual kidney function. The inserted PD catheter in the abdominal cavity of a patient, a system of bags: solution bag with dialysis fluid and an empty drainage bag for the effluent, and the transfer set (the tube that connects the PD catheter and the system of bags) are necessary for performing a CAPD (Figure 1).

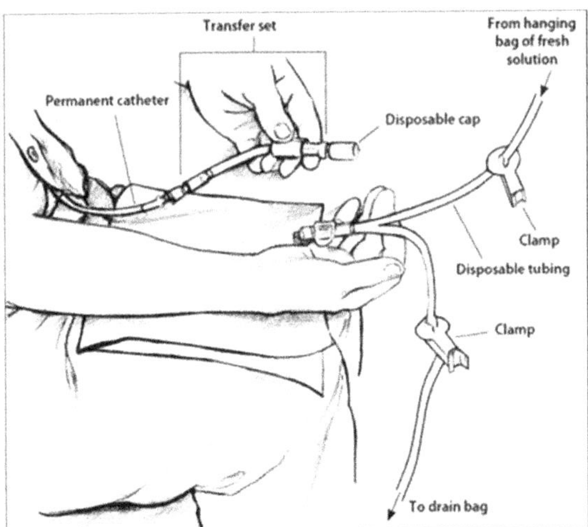


**Figure 1.** The external part of the PD catheter with transfer set that connects the PD catheter and the system of bags.

The patient manually connects the peritoneal catheter with the system of solution and drainage bag via a transfer set (Figure 1). The system ensures the drainage of the effluent from the abdominal cavity into the drainage bag, and the inflow of a new volume of dialysis fluid in the abdominal cavity of the patient (Figure 2). This process is called PD exchange.

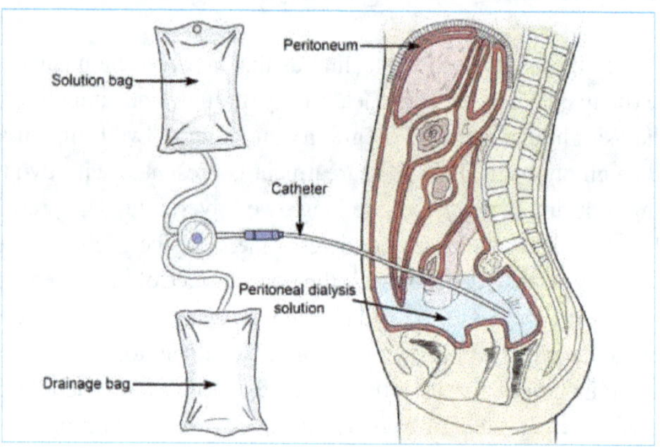


**Figure 2.** Presentation of a PD exchange.

The exchange process includes the following steps (Figure 1 and 2):

- The patient connects the transfer set connected to the PD catheter with the system of solution and empty (drainage) bag.
- The clamp holds the solution bag system closed. The clamp of the system connected to the empty bag and transfer set opens and allows the fluid to drain from the peritoneal cavity under the action of gravity into the empty bag. This process usually takes 10-15 minutes.
- The patient closes the clamp of the transfer set, opens the clamp of the solution bag, and allows the system of bags to be flushed of any contamination.
- Next, the patient closes the clamp on the system of drainage bag, and opens the clamp of the transfer set and the clamp of the solution bag, allowing dialysis fluid from the bag to flow through the PD catheter into the peritoneal cavity. This process usually takes 10-15 minutes.
- Finally, the patient manually disconnects the transfer set from the system of solution and drainage bag, and the transfer set is closed with a sterile cap (Figure 2).

## 5.2 Automated Peritoneal Dialysis (APD)

The mechanical device (cycler) is used for the instillation and drainage of the dialysis fluid from the peritoneal cavity. The exchanges with the cycler are made during the night (4 to 8-night cycles-exchanges), with the option for one or two long dwell daily exchanges.

APD regiments include:

- **Continuous cyclic peritoneal dialysis (CCPD):** reversal of CAPD, includes 3-4 exchanges during the night and 1-2 exchanges during the day (Figure 3).
- **Nocturnal intermittent PD (NIPD):** involves exchanges during the night, without daytime long exchanges (Figure 3).
- **Tidal peritoneal dialysis (TPD):** involves more exchanges during the night, without daytime long exchanges (Figure 3). During the exchange, only 50-80% of the dialysate is drained, and a new amount of dialysis fluid is instilled into the peritoneal cavity to lower the drainage discomfort and nighttime alarms. TPD is also the preferred treatment modality in patients with ascites as it allows a controlled outflow of fluid from the peritoneal cavity.
- **Continuous flow peritoneal dialysis (CFPD):** rapid, continuous movement of dialysis solution into and out of the peritoneal cavity. The potential application includes the treatment of acute kidney failure in intensive care units.

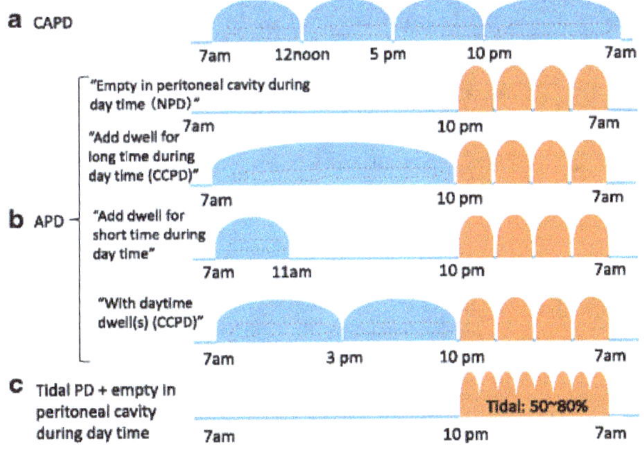


**Figure 3.** Different modalities of APD with various schedules of dwell time in peritoneal dialysis (PD). (Mizuno M, Suzuki Y, Sakata F et al. Which clinical conditions are most suitable for the induction of automated peritoneal dialysis? Ren Replace The 2016: 2, 46)

APD regimens allow for a large number of short-dwell exchanges during the night, and daily exchange, which improves the clearance of solutes and fluid. In the past, APD was reserved only for patients who were marked as "high-transporters", but recently, due to the lower cost of the cyclers, the APD is increasingly used in Europe and America. In APD there is no manual handling during the exchanges with a lower possibility for contamination and infection.

There are conflicting results in the literature about slower sodium clearance during APD due to short-dwell exchanges, with a higher risk of hypertension and faster decline in residual renal function in these patients. Cnossen TT et al. based on an analysis of 179 CAPD and 441 APD patients, showed that patient survival was not significantly different between APD and CAPD patients. The technique survival appeared to be higher in APD patients compared to CAPD patients, and could not be explained by differences in infectious complications. No difference in blood pressure control or decline in residual renal function was observed between the 2 modalities. In Mexico, Ramos Sanchez et al. performed a study on 139 CAPD and 98 APD patients to compare patient and technical survival as well as peritonitis rates in APD *vs.* CAPD. The APD *vs* CAPD patient survival for years 1, 2, and 3 was 82 *vs* 62%, 62 *vs* 49%, and 56 *vs* 42%, respectively (P=0.001). The technique survival for years 1, 2, and 3 was 76%, 56%, and 56% for APD and 65%, 47%, and 42% for CAPD patients. The only factor related to better survival was PD modality in favor of APD (P=0.001), but patients on APD were younger than those on CAPD. Peritonitis average rate was 1 episode per 34 patient-months on APD and 1 episode per 16 patient-months on CAPD. The possibility of a first peritonitis event during the first year was 21% on APD and 47% on CAPD (P=0.001). The results of a systematic review of randomized controlled trials performed by Rabindranath et al. showed that there were no differences in mortality, infectious complications, change of dialysis modality, mechanical complications, PD catheter removal, hospital admissions, dialysis adequacy,and residual renal function between patients on APD and CAPD.

# References

1. Brown EA, Davies SJ, Rutherford P, Meeus F, Borras M, Riegel W et al. Survival of functionally anuric patients on automated peritoneal dialysis: the European APD Outcome Study. J Am Soc Nephrol. 2003 Nov;14(11):2948-2957.
2. Peritoneal dialysis in National Institute of Diabetes and Digestive and Kidney Diseases (NIDDK), available at: https://www.niddk.nih.gov/health-information/kidney-disease/kidney-failure/peritoneal-dialysis.
3. Rabindranath KS, Adams J, Ali TZ, Daly C, Vale L, Macleod AM. Automated vs continuous ambulatory peritoneal dialysis: a systematic review of randomized controlled trials. Nephrol Dial Transplant. 2007 Oct;22(10):2991-2998.
4. Cnossen TT, Usvyat L, Kotanko P, van der Sande FM, Kooman JP, Carter M et al. Comparison of outcomes on continuous ambulatory peritoneal dialysis versus automated peritoneal dialysis: results from a USA database. Perit Dial Int. 2011 Nov-Dec;31(6):679-684.
5. Sanchez AR, Madonia C, Rascon-Pacheco RA. Improved patient/technique survival and peritonitis rates in patients treated with automated peritoneal dialysis when compared to continuous ambulatory peritoneal dialysis in a Mexican PD center. Kidney Int Suppl. 2008 Apr;(108):S76-80.
6. Vychytil A, Hörl WH. The role of tidal peritoneal dialysis in modern practice: A European perspective. Kidney Int Suppl. 2006 Nov;(103):S96-S103.
7. Kathuria, P., Twardowski, Z.J. (2023). Automated Peritoneal Dialysis. In: Khanna, R., Krediet, R.T. (eds) Nolph and Gokal's Textbook of Peritoneal Dialysis. Springer, Cham.
8. Amerling R, Winchester JF, Ronco C. Continuous flow peritoneal dialysis: update 2012. Contrib Nephrol. 2012;178:205-215.

## Chapter 6
## *Patient selection for peritoneal dialysis*

Only 5%-20% of patients on dialysis are treated with peritoneal dialysis in most countries worldwide, representing an underutilized dialysis modality. It is related to the availability and access to hemodialysis centers, or in some cases, patient preference for hemodialysis over peritoneal dialysis. In economically developed countries, the choice of peritoneal dialysis versus hemodialysis is sometimes a matter of patient preference, and sometimes due to lack of a hemodialysis unit that is easily accessible to the patient's home. In less economically developed countries, peritoneal dialysis may be the first choice, due to higher costs and difficulty accessing a hemodialysis center.

The Kidney Diseases Improving Global Outcome (KDIGO) recommended that all patients with GFR < 30 ml/min/1.73 m$^2$ (CKD stage 4/5) should be followed by a nephrologist. All patients with CKD stage 4/5 should be educated and concealed by a multidisciplinary team about all available modalities of kidney replacement therapy (KRT), including peritoneal dialysis, to make an informed decision for the treatment. The choice of the most appropriate KRT modality should be individualized and based on the patient's needs, motivation, abilities, and medical condition.

Blake PG et al. proposed the six key steps to optimize peritoneal dialysis and to identify all potential candidates for peritoneal dialysis among patients with kidney failure with the need to start dialysis treatment (Figure 1).

# The six steps to optimize incident PD

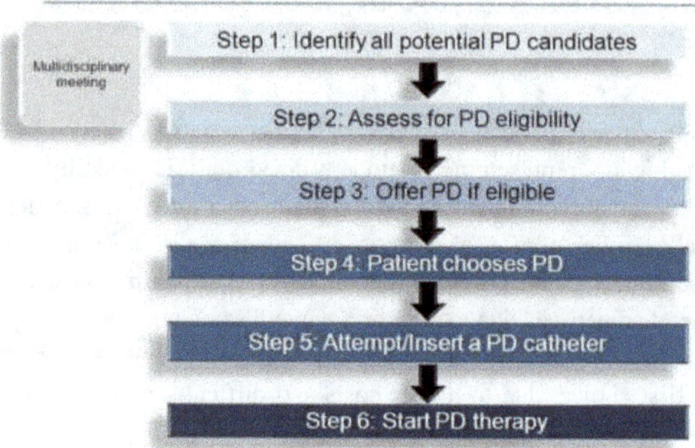


**Figure 1.** The six key steps to optimize the use of peritoneal dialysis. (Blake PG et al. Peritoneal dialysis and the process of modality selection. Perit Dial Int. 2013 May-Jun;33(3):233-241.)

The potential candidates for peritoneal dialysis are:

- Patients with kidney failure who started with dialysis (kidney transplantation is not planned or temporarily not available) and did not have any absolute contraindication for PD (based on the opinion of a nephrology team and informed decision of the patient)
- Patients treated with hemodialysis in a hemodialysis center
- Patients with more than 30 consecutive days of dialysis dependence, even if they have a presumed diagnosis of acute kidney injury
- Patients with a failed transplanted kidney graft requiring dialysis

The patients who started urgent hemodialysis treatment and were not previously followed by a nephrologist as patients with CKD, usually continue the KRT with hemodialysis. These patients started treatment with hemodialysis by default and most of them did not have an opportunity for education and selection of the most appropriate modality of KRT. All of these patients who were hemodialysis dependent for 30 consecutive days could be defined as a potential candidate for PD. They could participate in the education for KRT, with the possibility of an informed choice of the most appropriate modality of KRT.

## 6.1. Assessment for PD eligibility: contraindications and barriers

These factors should be evaluated for the patient's assessment for PD eligibility: patient's age, mental and physical capacity, comorbidities, history of surgical interventions, anticoagulation medication, distance to the PD unit, personal hygiene, social and economic status, lifestyle, presence/absence of caregivers of the patient and their willingness to participate in treatment. The most recent treatment guidelines (KDIGO 2012, NICE 2018, ERBP 2010) stated that only prerequisite for performing PD is a patient who is willing and motivated for PD, with intact peritoneal membrane.

The medical contraindications for the treatment with PD are:

- Major abdominal wall defects (surgically irreparable hernia, omphalocele, gastroschisis, diaphragmatic hernia, and bladder extrophy)
- Previous extensive abdominal surgeries with proved adhesions that could limit the dialysate flow
- Active ongoing bowel inflammation (active diverticulitis) and inflammatory bowel disease
- Morbid obesity
- Large abdominal aortic aneurysm
- Ostomies (ileostomies, colostomies)
- Residence of the patient without water in house
- Patients with blindness, or with physical or mental disabilities with the absence of assistance from caregivers

The barriers to the treatment with PD are factors that make the performing of PD a challenge, but they could be overcome if sufficient support is available to the patient:

- Previous extensive abdominal surgeries with possible adhesions: There is a growing number of patients with previous abdominal surgeries treated with PD. Abdominal surgery does not mean the presence of adhesions by default. In these cases, catheter insertion was performed by laparoscopic method which allows the detection of adhesions with adhesiolysis or omentopexy. Crabtree et al. reported long-term results of 436 laparoscopic PD catheter insertions, including 224 patients (57%) with a history of abdominal surgery. About 32% of the patients with prior abdominal surgery required adhesiolysis, and the number of previous surgeries was related to the occurrence of adhesions. The long-term catheter survival was unaffected by the history of adhesiolysis and surgery. Additionally, they discovered that past peritonitis and abdominal scars are not reliable indicators of the degree of adhesions and should not be utilized to determine a patient's eligibility for peritoneal dialysis.

- Cognitive impairment, psychiatric diseases (anxiety, depression), and impaired vision could be overcome by assisted PD.
- Elderly: Compared to HD, PD in elderly patients was associated with less risk for dialysis hypotension, fatigue, impaired myocardial function and arrhythmia, deterioration of cerebral function (secondary to ischemia), vascular access problems, and increased fall risk. Assisted PD might be rational in these patients.
- Diabetes mellitus: 60%–80% of glucose in glucose-containing PD solutions instilled into the peritoneal cavity is absorbed, corresponding to a daily intake of 100–300 g glucose, leading to hyperglycemia. The possible solution is the use of icodextrin and low glucose-containing solutions.
- Obesity: While in HD patients obesity (assessed by BMI) shows the so-called "obesity paradox", the study of Obi Y et al conducted on 15573 PD patients showed U-shaped distribution of mortality, and patients with a BMI of 30-35 $kg/m^2$ had the highest survival rate. According to the literature, peritoneal dialysis was not contraindicated in obese patients. Possible challenges included: increased risks of catheter leaks, exit-site infections, and a higher rate of peritonitis, which might be overcome with the use of upper abdominal or pre-sternal exit site PD catheter and closer follow-up of the patients.
- Polycystic kidney disease (PKD): Large kidneys with cysts, and very often the liver is also with cysts, occupy the abdominal cavity which could lead to inadequate PD. However, more recent evidence suggested that PKD patients have similar or even better survival on PD compared to HD. In these patients, it is reasonable to use lower volumes of dialysate and more frequent exchanges with APD.
- Cirrhosis: In cirrhotic patients, PD allowed anticoagulation-free dialysis, gradual fluid changes, improved hemodynamic stability, and increased caloric intake. Possible concerns included: increased risk for spontaneous bacterial peritonitis, catheter placement (ascites), greater peritoneal protein losses. Although HD remains the dominant modality, PD also could be a viable option for cirrhotic patients with kidney failure.
- Graft failure: Immunosuppression should be gradually reduced to preserve longer residual kidney function without raising the risk of peritonitis.
- Acute dialysis: According to KDIGO-AKI guidelines, patients with unstable hemodynamics, coagulopathy issues, inappropriate vessels for vascular access, increased intracranial pressure, and those who are inaccessible to continuous hemodialysis modalities for other reasons may be candidates for PD.

- Heart failure: PD provided well-tolerated and gentle fluid removal in patients with heart failure. Al-Hwiesh AK et al. conducted a study on 88 patients with heart failure randomized in two groups: 44 patients were treated with ultrafiltration HD and 44 were treated with tidal PD. After 90 days of follow-up, the PD group was superior to the  ultrafiltration HD group in terms of fluid loss, renal and cardiac recovery, and hospitalization rate.

## References


1. Blake PG, Quinn RR, Oliver MJ. Peritoneal dialysis and the process of modality selection. Perit Dial Int. 2013 May-Jun;33(3):233-241.
2. Eroglu E, Heimbürger O, Lindholm B. Peritoneal dialysis patient selection from a comorbidity perspective. Semin Dial. 2022 Jan;35(1):25-39.
3. Crabtree JH, Burchette RJ. Effective use of laparoscopy for long-term peritoneal dialysis access. Am J Surg. 2009 Jul;198(1):135-141.
4. Obi Y, Streja E, Mehrotra R, Rivara MB, Rhee CM, Soohoo M, et al. Impact of Obesity on Modality Longevity, Residual Kidney Function, Peritonitis, and Survival Among Incident Peritoneal Dialysis Patients. Am J Kidney Dis. 2018 Jun;71(6):802-813.
5. Al-Hwiesh AK, Abdul-Rahman IS, Al-Audah N, Al-Hwiesh A, Al-Harbi M, Taha A, et al. Tidal peritoneal dialysis versus ultrafiltration in type 1 cardiorenal syndrome: A prospective randomized study. Int J Artif Organs. 2019 Dec;42(12):684-694.

## Chapter 7

*Prescribing high-quality goal-directed peritoneal dialysis*

The International Society for peritoneal dialysis (ISPD) guidelines for small solute clearance and fluid removal in peritoneal dialysis were published in 2006. The Kt/V is a measure of urea clearance by dialysis: K = clearance (the amount of urea that dialysis can remove), t = time (the duration of treatment in minutes), and V = volume (volume of distribution of urea which is approximately equal to total body water in liters). The 2006 guidelines were: a weekly Kt/V urea > 1.7 especially if the PD patient is anuric, clearance of creatinine (CrCl) of 60 L/week/1.73m$^2$, and daily peritoneal ultrafiltration > 750 ml. The highlighted mark was that residual renal function (RRF) was associated with the survival of PD patients. These guidelines were released after several randomized controlled trials (RCTs) in the area of small solute clearance and outcomes of dialysis patients, published between 1999 and 2003.

The ADEMEX (ADEquacy of peritoneal dialysis in MEXico) study was a multicenter, prospective RCT to study the effects of increased peritoneal small solute clearance on the clinical outcomes of PD patients. It was performed in 24 dialysis centers in Mexico on 965 patients on CAPD. The patients were randomly assigned to a control or intervention group (in a 1:1 ratio). Patients in the control group continued to receive their preexisting CAPD prescriptions, which consisted of four daily exchanges with 2L of standard PD solution. The patients in the intervention group were treated with a modified PD regimen to achieve a peritoneal creatinine clearance (pCrCl) of 60 L/week/1.73 m$^2$. The first new prescription was based on body surface area (BSA), patients with BSA ≤1.78 m$^2$ received a prescription of four daily exchanges of 2.5L and patients with a BSA>1.78m$^2$ received a prescription of four daily exchanges of 3.0L. After 2 months, pCrCl was measured again. If the patients had reached the pCrCl target with the first prescription change, they continued with the same regimen to the end of the study, assured that they tolerated the increased fill volume. Patients who failed to reach the pCrCl target and with a tolerance of the increased fill volumes received a second modified prescription, which was also based on BSA. Patients with a BSA ≤1.78 m$^2$ received a second prescription of five daily exchanges of 2.5L, with the aid of an automated nighttime exchange device (Quantum; Baxter Healthcare Corp., Deerfield, IL), and patients with a BSA>1.78 m$^2$ received five daily exchanges of 3.0L with the aid of the same automated nighttime exchange device (Quantum). The minimal follow-up period was 2 years. There was no significant difference in total (renal plus peritoneal) CrCl between the control and intervention groups (61.8 ± 26.3 *vs.* 59.8 ± 20.2 L/week/1.73 m$^2$). There was also no significant difference in the total Kt/V values between the control and intervention groups (1.95 ± 0.67 *vs.* 1.93 ± 0.57). Patient survival was similar in the control and intervention groups, with an RR of death of 1.00 (95% CI:0.80-1.24). The control group exhibited a 1- year survival of 85.5% and a 2-year survival of 68.3%. The intervention groups exhibited a 1-year survival of 83.9% and a 2-year survival of 69.3%. Age, diabetes mellitus, serum albumin levels, and residual renal function were the factors significantly associated with the patient's survival.

In the open-labeled RCT, 320 new CAPD patients with baseline Kt/V<1.0 were recruited from six centers in Hong Kong and were randomized into three Kt/V target groups: group A with Kt/V target 1.5 to 1.7, group B with Kt/V target 1.7 to 2.0, and group C with Kt/V target >2.0. The overall 2-year patient survival was 84.9%. There was no significant difference in patient survival among the three groups (group A: 87.3%, group B: 86.1%, and group C: 81.5%).

The large observational cohort study in the United States on 1603 PD patients demonstrated that residual renal function, not the peritoneal clearance was associated with the patient survival.

The prospective multicenter study in the Netherlands on 413 PD patients demonstrated a significant 12% reduction in the mortality rate for each 1 mL/min/1.73m$^2$ increase in residual renal GFR. The 2-year patient survival was 84%. There was no significant effect of the peritoneal creatinine clearance on patient survival.

The 2019 update of the literature and revision of 2006 ISPD guidelines on targets for solute and fluid removal in PD patients was published in 2020. No new prospective intervention trials have been conducted about the small solute clearance with PD since the publication of the ISPD guidelines in 2006. The trials till 2019 were largely limited to a few prospective cohort studies and retrospective studies. These studies have consistently demonstrated that residual renal function was more often associated with the patient outcome than peritoneal clearance of small solutes, with no survival advantage with achievement of a weekly Kt/V>1.70.

The summary statements of 2019 update of the literature and revision of 2006 ISPD guidelines are:

- Residual renal function has been consistently demonstrated to be associated with outcomes in PD patients and therefore should be maintained

- Peritoneal clearance of small solutes has not been consistently associated with outcomes in PD patients
- There is no evidence that increasing weekly Kt/V>1.7–1.8 provides survival advantage
- There is evidence that a weekly Kt/V<1.7 is associated with increased morbidity
- In anuric people doing PD, a weekly Kt/V of at least 1.7 is recommended to prolong survival
- Peritoneal ultrafiltration (UF) is associated with overall and technique survival but no numerical target could be recommended
- Icodextrin is recommended to improve UF. There is no apparent risk of adverse side effects or impact on residual renal function
- In regions where icodextrin is not easily accessible, a manual daytime exchange may reduce negative UF in people on APD, particularly high transporters

The summary recommendations are:

- Measure residual renal function at baseline and at least once every 6 months in every PD patient.
- Measure residual renal clearance and peritoneal clearance in under-dialyzed or anuric PD patients at least once every 6 months.

In some PD centers, the healthcare providers were focused on achieving the small solute clearance targets suggested in the ISPD guidelines 2006 without taking into consideration the impact of increased dialysis exchanges or hours on a cycling machine on a person's quality of life. The need for a change in emphasis of care was the focus of discussion at the Kidney Disease Improving Global Outcomes (KDIGO) Controversies Conference on Dialysis Initiation, Modality Choice & Prescription in January 2018. At this meeting, it was proposed that there should be a change in terminology from 'adequate' dialysis to 'goal-directed' dialysis defined as 'using shared decision-making between the patient and care team to establish realistic care goals that will allow the patient to meet his/her own life goals and allow the clinician to provide individualized, high-quality PD care'. This approach would require multiple measures and goals to be considered when assessing the quality of dialysis, including the patient's symptoms, residual renal function, volume status, biochemical measures, nutritional status, cardiovascular function, small solute clearance, and sense of well-being and satisfaction. The Guideline Committee of the ISPD invited a group of globally representative nephrologists to compose new practice recommendations for prescribing high-quality, goal-directed PD in 2020.

The new practice key recommendations for prescribing high-quality, goal-directed PD are:

- PD should be prescribed using shared decision-making between the patient doing PD and the care team. The aim is to establish realistic care goals that (1) maintain quality of life for the PD patients as much as possible by enabling them to meet their life goals, (2) minimize symptoms and treatment burden while (3) ensuring high-quality care is provided.

The PD prescription should take into account the local country resources, the wishes, and lifestyle considerations of people needing treatment, including those of their families/caregivers, especially if assisting in their care. Several assessments should be used to ensure the delivery of high-quality PD care:

- Patient reports outcome measures – this is a measure of how a PD patient is experiencing life and his/her feeling of well-being. It should take into account the person's symptoms, and the impact of the dialysis regimen on the person's life, mental health, and social circumstances.
- Fluid status is an important part of dialysis delivery. Urine output and fluid removed by dialysis both contribute to maintaining good fluid status. Regular assessment of fluid status, including blood pressure and clinical examination, should be part of routine care.
- Removal of toxins should be estimated using a calculation called Kt/V urea and/or creatinine clearance (CrCl). Both are measures of the amount of dialysis delivered. There is no high-quality evidence regarding the need or benefit associated with the achievement of a specific target value for these measures. The residual renal function that continues to remove waste products and the remaining urine volume should be known for all PD patients. Management should focus on preserving residual renal function as long as possible.
- Nutrition status should be assessed regularly through evaluation of the patient's appetite, clinical examination, body weight measurements, and blood tests (potassium, bicarbonate, phosphate, albumin). Dietary intake of potassium, phosphate, sodium, protein, carbohydrate, and fat must be assessed and adjusted as well.
- For old, frail patients who have a poor prognosis but require dialysis treatment, there may be a life benefit from a reduced dialysis prescription to minimize the burden of treatment.
- In low and lower-middle-income countries, every effort should be made to comply with the framework of these statements, taking into account resource limitations.

- The principles of prescribing and assessing the delivery of high-quality PD to children are the same as for adults. In all cases, the PD prescription should be designed to meet the medical, mental health, social, and financial needs of the child and family.

At the most fundamental level, patients should have the choice of selecting CAPD or APD, with options for different fill volumes and a selection of dialysate solution (different concentrations of glucose or icodextrin-based solutions). The flexibility is even greater with APD, for which fill volumes could be increased in 100-mL increments, there are options about the number of exchanges overnight (generally 3-5) or during the day (generally 0-2), and different combinations of glucose-based solutions could be used overnight to optimize fluid removal. The observational studies comparing CAPD with APD have not shown a consistent effect of PD modality on health-related quality of life. Further options for PD include the use of urgent-start PD, incremental PD in individuals with significant residual renal function, assisted PD in people requiring support, and palliative PD in those nearing the end of life. Incremental peritoneal dialysis is prescribed in patients initiating PD with residual renal function, increasing the PD prescription, if and when residual renal function declines. Incremental PD prescription uses a lower dose of PD prescription compared to standard full-dose PD prescription. The lower dose of PD allows patients more time for life participation, less treatment burden, and a better quality of life..

Fluid status is an important part of high-quality dialysis treatment. Urine output and fluid removed by dialysis both contribute to maintaining the fluid status. Regular assessment of fluid status, including measurement of blood pressure (BP) and clinical examination (regular measurement of body weight, the volume of urine output, UF achieved by PD, presence of edema cruris and oedema pulmonum) should be part of routine care. The KDOQI workgroup supported the recommendation that the selection of PD modality (CAPD *vs.* APD) should be based on individual patient choice because there is no consistent evidence that one preserves residual renal function better than the other. Several clinical trials support the recommendation for the use of an angiotensin-converting enzyme inhibitor or angiotensin receptor blocker, loop diuretics, and neutral-pH low glucose degradation product PD solutions for the preservation of residual renal function. It is common practice to be cautious with the use of intravenous contrast and other potential nephrotoxins (aminoglycoside), although there were no studies that have shown an association of contrast administration with a sustained decrease in residual renal function in PD patients. Many PD patients are volume expanded, which contributes to hypertension and the development of left ventricular hypertrophy with a higher risk of cardiovascular mortality. Once-daily icodextrin should be considered as an alternative to hypertonic glucose solutions for long dwell (overnight exchange) in PD patients who are experiencing difficulties maintaining euvolemia due to insufficient peritoneal ultrafiltration, taking into account the individual's peritoneal transport state. Observational studies have demonstrated an association between higher daily PD ultrafiltration with lower mortality. Reducing dietary salt intake, maximizing urine volume, and optimizing peritoneal ultrafiltration are important components of management to reduce hypervolemia in PD patients. High-quality PD prescription should aim to achieve and maintain clinical euvolemia with preservation of residual renal function. There is also concern that aggressive PD ultrafiltration may result in a faster loss of residual renal function. Caution should be taken to avoid volume depletion and hypotension based on low-certainty evidence that this might adversely affect residual renal function. All efforts should be made to preserve residual renal function and peritoneal membrane function to maintain PD ultrafiltration for an extended period without the need to intensify PD prescription.

There is limited evidence for the benefits of better blood pressure (BP) control in PD patients. A study using the US Renal Data System database demonstrated higher mortality in patients with systolic BP < 111 mmHg but no effect of higher BP up to a systolic BP $\geq$ 180 mm Hg. The longer-term study from the United Kingdom demonstrated a lower risk for death with higher BP in the first 6 months of PD treatment, no effect till the 5th year of treatment, and then higher mortality after the 5th year of treatment. Currently, there is no evidence for a BP target in PD.

The KDOQI work group stressed that clinicians should follow up with patients closely for signs or symptoms if a weekly Kt/V < 1.7. If the patient's symptoms, nutrition, and volume status are all controlled, the PD prescription should not be changed for the sole purpose of reaching a small-solute clearance target. Patients who remain symptomatic despite a weekly Kt/V > 1.7 should have other dialysis and non-dialysis-related factors considered as possible contributing factors. A PD prescription with increasing dialysis dose might be indicated. Poor nutritional status and protein energy wasting should be evaluated when assessing the need to increase the dose of peritoneal dialysis. Factors that indicate the change of dialysate type or increase in PD prescription are uremic symptoms (increasing tiredness, loss of appetite, nausea, weight loss), symptomatic volume overload, poor nutritional status, hospitalization related to uremia or volume overload, a decline in urine volume, and biochemical features like hyperkaliemia, hyperphosphatemia, low plasma bicarbonate, rising urea, and creatinine (Table 1).

**Table 1**. Presentation of factors that indicate an increase in PD prescription or the change of dialysate type.

| Factor | Suggests need to change dialysate type or increase prescription |
| --- | --- |
| Clinical features | Uraemic symptoms, such as increasing tiredness, loss of appetite, nausea, weight loss (recognising there could be other causes of individual symptoms)<br>Symptomatic volume overload<br>Poor nutritional status or clinical features of protein-energy wasting<br>Hospitalization related to uraemia or volume overload<br>Poor or worsening school performance<br>Reduced energy level, physical activity or school attendance appropriate to child's age |
| Residual kidney function | Decline in urine volume and/or renal small solute removal |
| Biochemical features | Hyperkalaemia<br>Hyperphosphataemia<br>Low plasma bicarbonate<br>Worsening uraemia (rising urea and creatinine) |

(Brown EA et al International Society for peritoneal dialysis practice recommendations: Prescribing high-quality goal-directed peritoneal dialysis. Perit Dial Int. 2020 May;40(3):244-253)

# References


1. Lo WK, Bargman JM, Burkart J. Guideline on targets for solute and fluid removal in adult patients on chronic peritoneal dialysis. Perit Dial Int 2006; 26:520–522.
2. Paniagua R, Amato D, Vonesh E. Effects of increased peritoneal clearances on mortality rates in peritoneal dialysis: ADEMEX, a prospective, randomized, controlled trial. J Am Soc Nephrol 2002; 13(5):1307–1320.
3. Lo WK, Ho YW, Li CS, Wong KS, Chan TM, Yu AW et al. Effect of Kt/V on survival and clinical outcome in CAPD patients in a randomized prospective study. Kidney Int. 2003 Aug;64(2):649-656.
4. Diaz-Buxo JA, Lowrie EG, Lew NL, Zhang SM, Zhu X, Lazarus JM. Associates of mortality among peritoneal dialysis patients with special reference to peritoneal transport rates and solute clearance. Am J Kidney Dis. 1999 Mar;33(3):523-534.
5. Termorshuizen F, Korevaar JC, Dekker FW. The relative importance of residual renal function compared with peritoneal clearance for patient survival and quality of life: an analysis of the Netherlands Cooperative Study on the

Adequacy of Dialysis (NECOSAD)-2. Am J Kidney Dis 2003; 41(6):1293–1302.

6. Boudville N, de Moraes TP. 2005 Guidelines on targets for solute and fluid removal in adults being treated with chronic peritoneal dialysis: 2019 Update of the literature and revision of recommendations. Perit Dial Int. 2020 May; 40(3):254-260.

7. Chan CT, Blankestijn PJ, Dember LM. Dialysis initiation, modality choice, access, and prescription: conclusions from a kidney disease: improving global outcomes (KDIGO) controversies conference. Kidney Int 2019; 96: 37–47.

8. Brown EA, Blake PG, Boudville N, Davies S, de Arteaga J, Dong J, et al. International Society for Peritoneal Dialysis practice recommendations: Prescribing high-quality goal-directed peritoneal dialysis. Perit Dial Int. 2020 May;40(3):244-253.

9. Teitelbaum I, Glickman J, Neu A, Neumann J, Rivara MB, Shen J et al. KDOQI US Commentary on the 2020 ISPD Practice Recommendations for Prescribing High-Quality Goal-Directed Peritoneal Dialysis. Am J Kidney Dis. 2021 Feb;77(2):157-171.

10. Goldfarb-Rumyantzev AS, Baird BC, Leypoldt JK, Cheung AK. The association between BP and mortality in patients on chronic peritoneal dialysis. Nephrol Dial Transplant. 2005;20(8):1693-1701.

11. Udaya P. Udayaraj, Retha Steenkamp, Fergus J. Caskey, Chris Rogers, Dorothea Nitsch, David Ansell et al. Blood Pressure and Mortality Risk on Peritoneal Dialysis, American Journal of Kidney Diseases 2009; 53 (1): 70-78.

12. Wang AY, Brimble KS, Brunier G. ISPD cardiovascular and metabolic guidelines in adult peritoneal dialysis patients part I – assessment and management of various cardiovascular risk factors. Perit Dial Int 2015; 35(4):379–387.

13. Htay H, Johnson DW, Wiggins KJ. Biocompatible dialysis fluids for peritoneal dialysis. Cochrane Database Syst Rev 2018; 10: CD007554.

14. Rocco M, Soucie JM, Pastan S, et al. Peritoneal dialysis adequacy and risk of death. Kidney Int 2000; 58(1): 446–457.

*Chapter 8*
*Peritoneal equilibration test*


The peritoneal equilibration test (PET) is a semiquantitative assessment of peritoneal membrane transport function in patients on peritoneal dialysis. This test determines solute equilibration and peritoneal membrane transport rates by measuring dialysate to plasma ratio (D/P ratio) at specific times during dialysate dwell. The PET also measures ultrafiltration (UF) assessed by PD and residual renal function of the patient. Initial PET should be completed between 4 to 8 weeks after the commencement of maintenance PD therapy. The result from PET will assist the nephrologist in determining the best PD treatment suited for a patient. Repeat or subsequent PETs may be requested by the nephrologist if a change in peritoneal membrane transport function is suspected or when the nephrologist indicates an increase in PD prescription or change of dialysate type of renal replacement treatment.


## 8.1. Preparation for the PET

1. The day before PET, the APD patient will perform the dialysis using a PET-specific APD program with 2.5% PD fluid with no combination of different strengths of PD fluid. The 1.5% PD fluid could be used for patients unable to tolerate 2.5%. The APD treatment should be completed with the last fill for 4 – 8 hours before PET, with no drain before the PET. Dwell PD fluid for 4 – 8 hours before the test. The PET should be aborted if the dwell time for the last filled PD fluid is < 4 hours or > 8 hours.
2. The day before PET, the CAPD patient should dwell PD fluid for 8 – 12 hours before the test. The last CAPD exchange should be with 2.5% PD fluid, with a dwell time of 8 – 12 hours before the test, with no drain before PET. Use 1.5% PD fluid for patients unable to tolerate 2.5%. The PET should be aborted if the last CAPD exchange dwell time is < 8 hours or > 12 hours.

When the patient arrives at the PD department in the morning of the PET, the overnight dwell is drained while the patient is sitting up for at least 20 minutes.

## 8.2. Procedure

1. Before commencing PET, weigh the patient and record on the PET form;
2. Ensure overnight dwell time is appropriate (8 – 12 hours for CAPD patients or 4 – 8 hours for APD patients):

   a) Note the time the last evening bag was instilled for the CAPD patient or the time when the APD therapy ended;
   b) Note the start time of the first drain for PET;
   c) Calculate overnight dwell time and record on PET form.

3. Perform a CAPD exchange and use the same PD fluid strength used overnight to fill the patient:

   a) Drain out all PD effluent and record the weight of the drain bag on the PET form;
   b) Collect PD effluent sample from drain bag using aseptic technique ensuring all the key parts/sites are protected (aspirate 10 mL PD effluent and transfer to labeled specimen jar marked as "overnight PD fluid" for analysis of urea, creatinine, and glucose);
   c) Patient should lie down on a bed to start filling with PD fluid. Record the start time of filling with PD fluid on the PET form;
   d) Patient should roll from side to side every 2 minutes while filling with PD fluid. Record the end time of fill on the PET form;
   e) Collect another PD effluent sample using an aseptic technique ensuring all the key parts/sites are protected. Once the patient is full, drain out 200mL PD effluent into the empty PD fluid bag. Aspirate 10 mL PD effluent and transfer to patient labeled specimen jar marked as "0 hour PD fluid" for analysis of urea, creatinine, and glucose. Infuse the remaining 180 mL PD effluent back into the patient;
   f) Dwell PD fluid for 2 hours.

4. After the dwell of PD fluid for 2 hours:

   a) Collect the patient's blood, with a request form for serum albumin, urea, creatinine, and glucose test;
   b) Collect another PD effluent sample. Drain out 200mL PD effluent into the drain bag. Aspirate 10 mL PD effluent and transfer to patient labeled specimen jar marked as "2 hour PD fluid" for analysis of urea, creatinine,

and glucose. Infuse the remaining 180 mL PD effluent back into the patient;

   c) Dwell PD fluid for a further 2 hours (making it a total of 4 hours dwell time);

5. On the 4th hour of dwell, drain out all PD effluent and collect samples.

   a) For patients connecting to CAPD – use PD fluid strength as per the patient's regular PD regimen;
   b) Record the start time of drain on PET form;
   c) Drain out all PD effluent and record the weight of the drain bag on the PD form;
   d) Record the end time of drain on PET form;
   e) Shake drain bag thoroughly and aspirate 10 mL PD effluent and transfer to patient labeled specimen jar marked as "4 hour PD fluid" for analysis of urea, creatinine, and glucose";
   f) For CAPD or APD patients with day dwell – run PD fluid into the patient as required.

6. Send all 4 x patient-labeled specimen jars containing varying times of PD effluent sample (marked as overnight, 0 hour, 2 hour, and 4 hour PD fluid) with a patient's blood for analysis of urea, creatinine, and glucose.
7. The nurse will record blood and PD fluid test results on PET form and enter results in software for PET to calculate the peritoneal membrane transport type of the patient. The nephrologist should determine the optimal PD regimen for the patient.

## 8.3. Understanding the PET results

Once the PET samples are collected, both the serum and dialysate samples are analyzed for urea, creatinine, and glucose to calculate equilibration ratios. This is calculated as the dialysate-to-plasma or D/P ratio for urea and creatinine (Figure 1). This means that the concentration of urea or creatinine in the dialysate at each time point is divided by the concentration of urea or creatinine in the plasma ( serum) sample. For glucose, dividing the dialysate glucose concentration at each time point (D) by the glucose concentration in the 0-hour dialysate (Do) sample results in the equilibration ratios, glucose D/Do(Figure 1). The peritoneal membrane transport type of the patients is determined from these equilibration ratios.

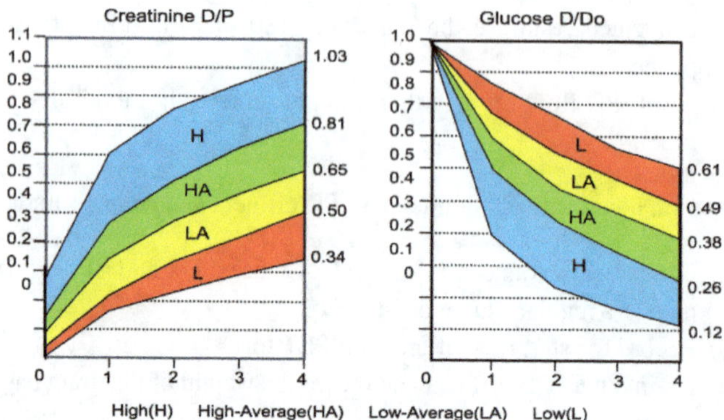


**Figure 1.** Calibration curves for peritoneal equilibrium test, for determining the transport types of peritoneal membrane. (Ito Y, Tawada M, Yuasa H, Ryuzaki M. New Japanese Society of Dialysis Therapy Guidelines for peritoneal dialysis. Contrib Nephrol. 2019;198:52-61)

The outer edges of the blue and red areas represent the maximum and minimums for the group. The patients are categorized based on the 4-hour D/P creatinine and D/Do glucose ratios. For example, if the 4-hour D/P creatinine is 0.59 and the 4-hour D/Do glucose is 0.47, the patient would be classified as a low-average transporter (LA).

The high (H) and high-average (HA) transporters equilibrate rapidly (Figure 1). This means their transports for urea and creatinine are fast, but it also means that they lose the glucose gradient rapidly with reabsorption of the water during the dwell with limited ultrafiltration. These patients would do best with more frequent exchanges with shorter dwells to avoid reabsorption. The best treatment for high transporters is APD and icodextrin should be considered for daytime dwell. If the patient has a good residual renal function, it might be possible to have a dry day period. High-average transporters might be treated with APD or CAPD.

The low (L) and low-average (LA) transporters equilibrate slowly. This means their transports for urea and creatinine are slower, which results in good ultrafiltration with minimal reabsorption of water, even for a long day dwell. They may require longer dwells with higher-volume exchanges to get adequate clearance of solutes. For the low-average transporter with good residual function, treatment with CAPD or APD is recommended, meaning continuous 24-hour therapy with no dry day periods. If the patient does not have significant residual function, high-dose CAPD with larger-dwell volumes will be necessary. The best treatment for low transporters is high-dose CAPD with larger-dwell volumes.

# References


1. Blake PG, Bargman JM, Brimble KS, Davison SN, Hirsch D, McCormick BB, et al. Canadian Society of Nephrology Work Group on Adequacy of Peritoneal Dialysis. Clinical Practice Guidelines and Recommendations on Peritoneal Dialysis Adequacy 2011. Perit Dial Int. 2011 Mar-Apr;31(2):218-239.
2. Brown EA, Blake PG, Boudville N, Davies S, de Arteaga J, Dong J, et al. International Society for Peritoneal Dialysis practice recommendations: Prescribing high-quality goal-directed peritoneal dialysis. Perit Dial Int. 2020 May;40(3):244-253.
3. Lo WK, Bargman JM, Burkart J, Krediet RT, Pollock C, Kawanishi H, et al. ISPD Adequacy of Peritoneal Dialysis Working Group. Guideline on targets for solute and fluid removal in adult patients on chronic peritoneal dialysis. Perit Dial Int. 2006 Sep-Oct;26(5):520-522.
4. Gokal R, Chan CK. Adequacy targets in peritoneal dialysis. J Nephrol. 2004 Nov-Dec;17(8):S55-67.
5. Ito Y, Tawada M, Yuasa H, Ryuzaki M. New Japanese Society of Dialysis Therapy Guidelines for Peritoneal Dialysis. Contrib Nephrol. 2019;198:52-61.

*Chapter 9*
## *Noninfectious complications of peritoneal dialysis*

Non-infectious complications of peritoneal dialysis (NICPD) have a significant impact on the quality and technical failure of peritoneal dialysis. NICPD could be a result of the placement and maintenance of the PD catheter, dialysate-induced increase in intra-abdominal pressure, and the metabolic effects of glucose from dialysis solutions (Table 1).

**Table 1.** Noninfectious complications of peritoneal dialysis

| **Catheter-related noninfectious complications** | **Complications related to increased intra-abdominal pressure** |
|---|---|
| Perioperative complications | Hernias |
| Impaired flow through the catheter | Pleural-peritoneal leak (hydrothorax) |
| Infusion/drainage pain | Scrotal leak |
| Pericatheter leak | Back pain |
| **Metabolic noninfectious complications** | **Miscellaneous** |
| Hyperglycemia and metabolic syndrome | Hemoperitoneum |
| Hypokalemia | Encapsulating peritoneal sclerosis |
| Hyponatremia and hypernatremia | |
| Protein loss (albumin) | |

(McCormick et al. Noninfectious Complications of PD: Implications for Patient and Technique Survival. Journal of the American Society of Nephrology 18(12): 3023-3025)

The study by Ahbap E et al. performed on 262 PD patients, showed that during the 20-year follow-up period, 185 (71%) patients experienced 382 NICPD episodes, and 26 patients (9.9%) were switched to maintenance hemodialysis because of NICPD. PD catheter outflow failure was the most common NICPD (total 97 episodes, 25%), with required catheter revision in 23 patients and PD discontinuation in 12 patients. The authors found that prior HD treatment and male gender were independent risk factors for NICPD and catheter-related complications (OR 2.076, P=0.037, and OR

65

1.797, P=0.042, respectively). Early start with PD (higher GFR) was associated with a lower risk for the development of NICPD (OR 0.393, P=0.013). Chan R et al. demonstrated that NICPD occurred within 30 days of initiation of PD, were associated with a higher risk of overall mortality (HR 1.71, 95%CI:1.21-2.44), PD discontinuation (HR 1.84, 95%CI: 1.41-2.41), and first catheter failure (HR 2.89, 95%CI: 2.28-3.66). The metabolic effects of the glucose from the dialysate could increase the cardiovascular risk of PD patients. The early recognition and management of NICPD could be crucial for the improvement of the survival and longer duration of PD.

## 9.1 Catheter-related noninfectious complications

PD-catheter associated mechanical problems are the most common noninfectious complications and account for nearly 20% of transfers to HD. The choice of an appropriate type of PD catheter, adequate implantation technique, and appropriate postoperative care are strategies that could prevent catheter malfunction. The catheter-related noninfectious complications are presented with:

- **Perioperative complications:**
    - **Intestinal perforation**: occurred in less than 1% of PD patients, usually in those with the need for urgent start of PD. The manifestation of intestinal perforation occurs a few hours after the catheter insertion. Feculent dialysate and diarrhea occurring after dialysate instillation should be an indication for an immediate CT scan of the abdomen and a consultation with a surgeon.
    - **Bladder perforation**: extremely rare, described in case reports. The patients present with a sudden increase in urine volume, urinary incontinence with dialysate inflow, and bladder discomfort.
    - **Bleeding:** mild relatively common complication, but severe bleeding is encountered in only 1% to 5% of procedures. Pericannular bleeding close to the exit site is the most common form and is managed with manual pressure, additional suturing, and local administration of epinephrine or desmopressin acetate. Rectus sheath hematoma also has been observed after PD catheter insertion.
- **Impaired flow through the catheter:**
    - **Inflow failure:** the dialysate solution won't leak into the peritoneum through the catheter.

- **Outflow failure:** the drainage volume in the empty bag is significantly less than the previously installed volume of dialysate in the peritoneum through the catheter. There is no sign of leakage.

The PD catheter's impaired flow could be caused by constipation, tissue attachment and entrapment of the catheter, internal luminal catheter obstruction by fibrin or blot clots, external compression of the catheter tip, and inadequate placement and/or migration of the catheter. External compression of the PD catheter tip  might be caused by constipation or bladder distension which obstructs the side holes of the catheter and impairs the draining of dialysate. Laxatives are used for the treatment of constipation. Some cases of external PD catheter compression might be caused by omental wrapping or ensnaring by adhesions within the peritoneal cavity. The management is using laparoscopic techniques for adhesiolysis and omentectomy.

- **Infusion/drainage pain:** when the PD catheter is placed too deep in the pelvis some patients might experience pain or discomfort during the infusion and/or draining of the dialysate. There is inadequate evacuation of dialysate fluid as organs in the pelvis are "sucking" to the catheter tip generating contact and irritation against the parietal peritoneum. In these cases, the catheter replacement is required.
- **Pericatheter leak:** pericatheter leak might occur early (within 30 days) or late after PD catheter placement. Early pericatheter leak is usually seen in patients with an urgent start of PD because the catheter exit site is not fully healed. In these cases, it is recommended to use a small in-flow volume of PD solution and to avoid activities that increase the intraabdominal pressure. Delaying the start of PD for two weeks after PD catheter insertion ("break-in period") could minimize the risk of pericatheter leak. In severe cases of leakage, the patient must be temporarily switched to hemodialysis. The treatment includes a new tight purse string suture around the deep cuff of the PD catheter within the rectus muscle and prophylactic antibiotics. Late pericatheter leak presents with occult tunnel infections or pericatheter hernia when the deep cuff of the PD catheter was positioned incorrectly in the midline fascia or outside the rectus muscle. Catheter revision and replacement are required in these patients.
- **Catheter cuff extrusion:** catheter cuff extrusion occurs as a consequence of repeated exit-site infections, substantial weight loss, or excessive catheter bending during the placement. The patients are treated with the cuff-shaving procedure (removal of the extruded outer cuff with the use of blunt forceps) or catheter removal.

## 9.2 Complications related to increased intra-abdominal pressure

The dialysate-induced increase in intra-abdominal pressure (IPP) in PD patients was associated with increased morbidity, mortality, and failure of PD technique with transfer to hemodialysis treatment. The intra-abdominal pressure is usually caused by high volumes of installed PD solution. It could cause discomfort, fullness, sleep disturbances, hemodynamic, and respiratory alterations. Also, it could predispose patients to hydrothorax (pleural-peritoneal leak), peritoneal-vaginal hydrocele, genital edema (scrotal leak), hernia, gastroesophageal reflux, hemorrhoids, and back pain. Patients with pleural-peritoneal leak have shortness of breath, reduced exchange volume, and new unilateral pleural effusion, with an indication for diagnostic and/or therapeutic pleural aspiration. The long-term management of a pleuroperitoneal leak depends on its severity. With conservative treatment, temporary transfer to hemodialysis treatment from six weeks to three months, the success rate for re-starting PD is approximately 50%. High IPP was also associated with ultrafiltration failure, more frequent episodes of peritonitis with intestinal bacteria, and increased production of endothelin, related to the long-term deterioration of the peritoneum. The factors that create IPP are residual volume of previously infused dialysate, newly infused volume of dialysate, body position (sitting > standing > lying down), physical activity, and BMI (obesity is associated with higher IPP). In stable adult PD patients with infused dialysate with volume of 2 L, a measured IPP of 10–16 cmH$_2$O on the mid-axillary line was considered acceptable IPP. Higher IPP values were associated with symptoms. The measurement of IPP could optimize the use of an appropriate volume of dialysate to achieve the highest clearance of solutes with avoiding the IPP-related complications.

## 9.3 Metabolic noninfectious complications

The most commonly used dialysate solutions contain a carbohydrate (glucose) as an osmotically active agent. Transperitoneal absorption of glucose could cause systemic metabolic changes such as weight gain, hyperglycemia, hyperinsulinemia, metabolic syndrome, new-onset diabetes mellitus, and dyslipidemia. The amount of absorbed glucose from dialysate depends on the peritoneal membrane permeability. High transporters could absorb glucose more quickly compared to low transporters. High transporters could absorb up to 80% of the glucose from dialysate into blood. Glucose absorption from dialysate could be calculated by using the following equation: Glucose absorption (g) = [glucose concentration of infused dialysate x infused dialysate volume] – [glucose concentration in drained dialysate (g/L) x drained dialysate volume]. There is less glucose absorption in APD compared to CAPD because APD has more cycles with shorter dwell time of dialysate.

Standard PD solutions do not contain potassium, and a CAPD regimen of 8L eliminates approximately 40 mmol of potassium daily, which is about the normal potassium intake. Thus, CAPD patients are susceptible to hypokalemia ($K^+$ < 3.5 mmol/L), if they continue the low-potassium diet from their pre-dialysis period. Hypokalemia has been identified as a risk factor for peritonitis and death in chronic PD patients.

Hyponatremia (dilutional or translocational as a result of extracellular water shifting due to high serum glucose) and hypernatremia (rapid ultrafiltration by using hypertonic solution) could be noted in PD patients. Protein loss through the peritoneal membrane might be significant and PD patients usually have lower serum albumin levels compared to HD patients.


## 9.4 Miscellaneous noninfectious complications

Hemoperitoneum could be caused by the PD catheter placement or other procedures, infectious processes, vascular or intra-abdominal organs, or obstetric or gynecological causes. Only 2 mL of blood in a 1-liter peritoneal fluid drainage bag could change the color of the fluid. The treatment is based on the treatment of the underlying cause of hematoperitoneum.

Encapsulating peritoneal sclerosis (EPS) is a rare but serious complication of long-term PD. EPS is characterized by peritoneal thickening and fibrosis, resulting in the formation of a fibrous cocoon, which could encapsulate the bowel, leading to intestinal obstruction. The pathogenesis of EPS includes damage of the peritoneal membrane from glucose during long-term PD and from episodes of peritonitis in genetically susceptible patients. Medical management of EPS includes the use of corticosteroids and/or tamoxifen. Steroids act by decreasing inflammation and the development of fibrin deposition.

**References**

1. McCormick, Brendan B Bargman, Joanne M. Noninfectious Complications of PD: Implications for Patient and Technique Survival. Journal of the American Society of Nephrology. 18(12): 3023-3025.
2. Oza-Gajera BP, Abdel-Aal AK, Almehmi A. Complications of Percutaneous Peritoneal Dialysis Catheter. Semin Intervent Radiol. 2022 Feb.18;39(1):40-46.
3. Kennedy C, Bargman, J.M. (2023). Noninfectious Complications of Peritoneal Dialysis. In: Khanna, R., Krediet, R.T. (eds) Nolph and Gokal's Textbook of Peritoneal Dialysis. Springer, Cham.
4. Ahbap E, Mazi EE, Basturk T, Sakaci T, Aykent MB, Unsal A. Peritoneal dialysis related non-infectious complications: A single-center experience over 20 years. Clin Nephrol. 2023 Jul; 100(1):19-26.
5. Chan R, Walker RJ, Samaranayaka A, Schollum J. Long-term impact of early non-infectious complications at the initiation of peritoneal dialysis. Perit Dial Int. 2023 Jan;43(1):53-63.
6. Bargman JM. Complications of peritoneal dialysis related to increased intraabdominal pressure. Kidney Int Suppl. 1993 Feb;40:S75-80.
7. Pérez Díaz V, Sanz Ballesteros S, Hernández García E, Descalzo Casado E, Herguedas Callejo I, Ferrer Perales C. Intraperitoneal pressure in peritoneal dialysis. Nefrologia. 2017 Nov-Dec; 37(6):579-586.
8. Stephen G, Alfred N, George L, Stone WJ. Hemoperitoneum: A Red Flag in CAPD. Peritoneal Dialysis International. 1985; 5(1):42-44.
9. Moinuddin Z, Summers A, Van Dellen D, Augustine T, Herrick SE. Encapsulating peritoneal sclerosis-a rare but devastating peritoneal disease. Front Physiol. 2015 Jan 5;5:470.

## 10.1. Peritonitis

Peritoneal dialysis-associated peritonitis is the most serious complication of PD associated with frequent hospitalizations of patients (5.9 hospital admissions per 100 patient-years, according to the  US Renal Data Systems report year 2022), technical failure, and patient's mortality. Peritonitis was the leading cause of transfer from peritoneal dialysis to hemodialysis (technical failure). In 2022, the International Society for Peritoneal Dialysis (ISPD) published the latest update of ISPD guidelines for peritonitis. The diagnosis of peritonitis associated with PD requires the presence of at least two of the following criteria:

- abdominal pain and cloudy dialysis effluent;
- dialysis effluent white cell count > 100/μL or > 0.1 X $10^9$/L (after a dwell time of at least 2 h), with > 50% polymorphonuclear leukocytes (PMN);
- positive dialysis effluent culture.

The rate of peritonitis should be reported as the number of episodes of peritonitis per patient-year of treatment with peritoneal dialysis. Patient-year is defined as the number of years on PD, starting from the time on which the first PD exchange was performed. The new recommended target for the overall peritonitis rate should be no more than 0.40 episodes per year. The percentage of patients free of peritonitis per unit time should be targeted at > 80% per year. The proportion of culture-negative peritonitis should be less than 15% of all peritonitis episodes. The peritonitis associated with PD is classified according to the cause, the timing of previous episode and outcome (Table 1).

**Table 1:** ISPD definitions for cause-specific, time-specific, and outcome-specific peritonitis.

| Cause-specific peritonitis | |
|---|---|
| Culture-positive peritonitis | diagnosis of peritonitis according to organisms identified on the culture of dialysis effluent |
| Culture-negative peritonitis | peritonitis is diagnosed with the presence of symptoms or cloudy effluent and the presence of white cell count > 100/μL in effluent, but no organism is identified on the culture of dialysis effluent |

| | |
|---|---|
| Catheter-related peritonitis | peritonitis that occurs within 3 months of the PD catheter infection with the same organism isolated from the exit site or from a tunnel collection of the PD catheter |
| Enteric peritonitis | peritonitis arising from inflammation, perforation, or ischemia of intraabdominal organs |
| **Time-specific peritonitis** | |
| Pre-PD peritonitis | Peritonitis occurs after PD catheter insertion and before the commencement of PD treatment. It is believed that this form of peritonitis is underestimated, and the incidence of pre-PD peritonitis was reported to be up to 4.2% of new patients on PD |
| PD-related peritonitis | Peritonitis occurring after PD commencement |
| PD catheter insertion-related peritonitis | An episode of peritonitis that occurs within 30 days of PD catheter insertion |
| **Outcome-specific definitions of peritonitis** | |
| Medical cure | Complete resolution of peritonitis without complications such as relapse/recurrent peritonitis, catheter removal, transfer to hemodialysis for more 30 days, or death |
| Refractory | Peritonitis with persistently cloudy effluent or persistent effluent leukocyte count > $100/\mu L$ after 5 days of appropriate antibiotic therapy. |
| Recurrent | Peritonitis episode that occurs within 4 weeks of completion of therapy of a prior episode but with a different organism. |
| Relapsing | Peritonitis episode that occurs within 4 weeks of completion of therapy of a prior episode with the same organism. Culture-negative peritonitis followed by peritonitis from a specific organism. Peritonitis from a specific organism followed by culture-negative peritonitis. |
| Repeat | Peritonitis episode that occurs after 4 weeks of completion of therapy of a prior episode with the same organism |

Globally, peritonitis rates vary significantly within PD units in various countries. Peritoneal Dialysis Outcomes and Practice Patterns Study (PDOPPS) was an international multicentric study that evaluated the peritonitis rates in 7051 adult PD patients in 209 facilities from seven countries. Overall peritonitis rates, in episodes per patient-year of treatment , were 0.40 in Thailand, 0.38 in the United Kingdom, 0.35 in Australia/New Zealand, 0.29 in Canada, 0.27 in Japan, and 0.26 in the United States. Except in Thailand, peritonitis episodes with Gram-positive microorganisms predominated in the rest of the analyzed countries. Median length of hospitalization was less than 1 week in all countries except in Japan with median lenght of 18 days and Thailand with median lenght of 11 days. There was a concomitant exit-site infection in 6% to 20% of peritonitis episodes. Lower peritonitis rates were observed in the facilities with a greater proportion of patients using APD, facilities that used antibiotics at catheter insertion, and facilities with PD training duration of 6 or more days. Lower peritonitis risk was detected in facilities that used topical exit-site mupirocin or aminoglycoside ointment, but without statistical significance. Marshall RM et al. performed a systematic review of peritoneal dialysis-related peritonitis rates over time in 33 countries. PD peritonitis rates were decreasing steadily over time, from 0.6 episodes per patient-year in 1992 to 0.3 in 2019.

Patients with PD-related peritonitis usually present with cloudy dialysis effluent, diffuse abdominal pain, and abdominal tenderness on palpation. Any discharge from the exit site and erythema, tenderness, and the presence of fluid collections along the PD catheter tunnel might be indicative of catheter exit-site or tunnel infection. When caused by Gram-negative enteric bacteria, peritonitis typically presents with more severe clinical signs and symptoms, such as fever, intense abdominal pain, nausea, vomiting, and diarrhea. In patients suspected of peritonitis, ISPD recommended PD effluent shold be tested for cell count, differential count, Gram stain, and culture. PD patients presenting with cloudy effluent are presumed to have peritonitis and should be treated with antibiotics until the diagnosis is confirmed or excluded.

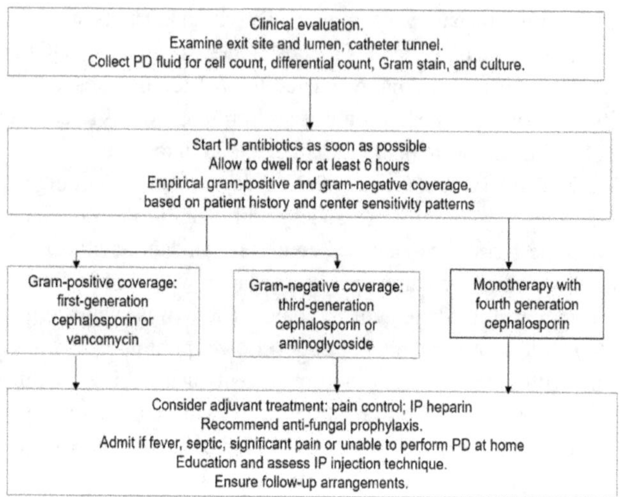


**Figure 1.** ISPD algorithm for initial management of PD patients suspected with peritonitis (ISPD peritonitis guideline recommendations: 2022 update on prevention and treatment)

Performing Gram staining, microscopic examination, and culture of PD effluent provided a bacteriological diagnosis in over 75% of cases with peritonitis in three days. When cultures remain negative after 3–5 days of incubation, PD effluent should be sent for repeat cell count with differential count, and to be cultured for fungus and mycobacteria. The peripheral blood cultures are not obligatory unless the patient has signs of systemic sepsis or is on immune-suppression therapy. The antibiotic therapy should be initiated after the collection of dialysis effluent for analysis without waiting for the results of laboratory testing (Figure 1). ISPD recommends that empirical antibiotic regimens be center-specific and cover both Gram-positive (first-generation cephalosporin or vancomycin) and Gram-negative organisms (third-generation cephalosporin or an aminoglycoside). Intraperitoneal (IP) administration is the preferred route of application of antibiotics unless the patient has features of systemic sepsis. The antibiotics are dilutied in the PD solution and instilled in to the peritoneum for a minimum duration of 6 hours. The dose of antibiotics should be properly adjusted to the body weight and residual renal function. Heparin dose of 500 units per L dialysate IP could be added to patients with peritonitis to prevent obstructing the PD catheter with fibrin. Urokinase could be used for the treatment of biofilm in refractory or relapsing peritonitis. Extensive peritoneal lavage did not improve the rate of complete medical cure. Due to increased peritoneal permeability during peritonitis, the use of Icodextrin should be considered to achieve better ultrafiltration. The treatment of peritonitis in patients with APD is a special challenge because of the frequent exchanges that lead to shorter antibiotic half-lives and inadequate serum and dialysate drug concentrations throughout 24 hours. There was an insufficient evidence on whether patients on APD should be temporarily switched to CAPD during treatment of peritonitis. The antibiotic therapy should be adjusted once microbiological results and sensitivities are known. PD catheter should be removed in a refractory peritonitis episode defined as failure of the PD effluent to clear after 5 days of appropriate antibiotics. Longer antibiotic treatment without removal of the catheter could be considered in patients where the dialysis effluent white cell count is decreasing toward normal. Fungal peritonitis is an indication for immediate removal of the PD catheter. For relapsing, recurrent, or repeat peritonitis episodes, it is recommended timely PD catheter removal and reinsertion after the culture of the PD effluent has become negative and the PD effluent white cell count is below 100/μL, in the absence of concomitant exit site or tunnel infection.

**Table 2.** Cause-specific peritonitis: recommended antibiotics and duration of treatment (ISPD peritonitis guideline recommendations 2022: update on prevention and treatment)

| Identified microorganism | Recommended antibiotic (usually effective antibiotic) | Duration of treatment |
|---|---|---|
| *Coagulase-negative Staphylococcus* | IP cephalosporin or vancomycin | 2 weeks |
| *Methicillin-sensitive Staphylococcus aureus* | IP first-generation cephalosporin | 3 weeks |
| *Methicillin-resistant Staphylococcus aureus* | IP vancomycin<br><br>oral rifampicin | 3 weeks |
| *Streptococcus* | IP cefazolin | 2 weeks |
| *Corynebacterium* | IP cefazolin<br><br>IP vancomycin (for *Corynebacterium jeikeium*) | 2 weeks |
| *Enterococcus* | IP ampicillin and vancomycin | 3 weeks |
| *Vancomycin-resistant Enterococcus* | oral or intravenous linezolid<br><br>or IP daptomycin or teicoplanin | 3 weeks |

| | | | |
|---|---|---|---|
| *Pseudomonas* | two IP antibiotics with different mechanisms (ceftazidime or cefepime + amikacin or tobramycin or gentamicin) | | 3 weeks |
| *Acinetobacter* | oral ciprofloxacin or oral trimethoprim/sulfamethoxazole or IP meropenem or aminoglycoside or colistin +/- ampicillin/sulbactam | | 3 weeks |
| *Stenotrophomonas maltophilia* | 2 effective antibiotics, one of them being trimethoprim-sulfamethoxazole | | 3 weeks |
| *Enteric gram-negative peritonitis* | Not specified | IP ceftazidime | 3 weeks |
| | | IP cefepime | |
| | ESBL producing | IP meropenem | |
| | Beta-lactamase producing | IP cefepime or meropenem or oral ciprofloxacin | |
| | Carbapenemase-producing Enterobacterales (CPE) | Type of carbapenemase with expert advise | |
| *Fungal peritonitis* | Immediate catheter removal with treatment: IV fluconazole for Candida albicans, other Candida organisms require an echinocandin (caspofungin, micafungin or anidulafungin) or voriconazole.<br><br>Aspergillus require: intravenous amphotericin B or voriconazole, posaconazole or isavuconazole | | treatment at least 2 weeks after catheter removal |
| *Mycobacterium tuberculosis* | four anti-tuberculous drugs for a total of 2 months, followed by two drugs (isoniazid and rifampicin) given for at least a total of 12 months | | |
| Non-tuberculous mycobacterial peritonitis | catheter removal with two agents to which the isolate is susceptible for a minimum of 6 weeks | | |

**Prevention of peritonitis**

- Systemic prophylactic antibiotics should be administered before catheter placement.
- Daily topical application of antibiotic cream or ointment to the catheter exit site and avoidance of mechanical stress may be useful to lower exit-site infection and peritonitis rate.
- PD patients should seek help from the PD center in case of "dry contamination" (contamination outside of a closed PD system) and "wet contamination" (contamination with an open system). Prophylactic antibiotics were recommended for wet contamination.
- Antibiotic prophylaxis and drainage of PD dialysate were advised before colonoscopy and invasive gynecological procedure.
- Optimal PD training and retraining program.
- Pets are not allowed in the room where PD exchange takes place, and where dialysis tubing, equipment, and machine are stored.
- Avoidance and treatment of hypokalemia and avoidance of use of histamine-2 receptor antagonists may reduce the risk of peritonitis.
- Anti-fungal prophylaxis be co-prescribed whenever PD patients receive an antibiotic course, regardless of the indication for that antibiotic course.


## 10.2. PD catheter-related infection

Peritoneal dialysis (PD) catheter-related infections are important risk factors for catheter loss and peritonitis. In 2023, International Society for Peritoneal Dialysis (ISPD) published the latest update of ISPD catheter-related infection guidelines (Table 3). A new target for the overall PD catheter-related infection rate should be no more than 0.40 episodes per year at risk. The proportion of PD catheter insertion-related infection should be less than 5% of all catheters inserted.

**Table 3.** ISPD definition for type, cause, and outcome of PD catheter-related infections

| Type of catheter-related infection | |
| --- | --- |
| Exit site infection | presence of purulent discharge, with or without erythema of the skin at the exit site of the catheter |
| Tunnel infection | presence of inflammation (erythema, swelling, tenderness, or induration) with or without ultrasonographic evidence of a fluid collection anywhere along the catheter tunnel |
| **Cause-specific catheter-related infection** | |
| Culture-positive | Most often isolated organisms: *Diphtheroid* (20.5%), *Staphylococcus aureus* (13.6%), *Pseudomonas aeruginosa* (13.6%), and *Fungus* (9.1%) |
| Culture-negative | exit site infection is diagnosed using the criteria above, but no organism is identified on the culture of the exit site swab |
| **PD catheter insertion-related exit site and/or tunnel infection** | |
| An episode of exit site infection/tunnel infection that occurs within 30 days of PD catheter insertion | |
| **Outcome-specific definitions of catheter-related infection** | |
| Refractory infection | failure to respond after 2 weeks of effective antibiotic therapy, and appropriately intensified exit site care, or 3 weeks for infection due to Pseudomonas species |
| Infection-related catheter removal | Removal of PD catheter due to refractory infection that does not respond to standard antibiotic treatment or surgical procedures |

When there is purulent discharge from the catheter exit site, a culture swab and Gram stain should be obtained (Figure 2). Careful inspection of the exit site and the tunnel of the catheter should be done, as well as milking of the track wound in case of suspected tunnel infection. Ultrasound examination and detection of purulent collections might be helpful in tunnel infection. Daily cleaning and monitoring of the exit site of the catheter is required for local treatment and monitoring of the clinical response. ISPD 2023 recommended empiric oral antibiotic treatment of exit site infections with appropriate coverage for *S. aureus* such as first-generation cephalosporin or anti-staphylococcal penicillin. If the patient has a prior history of infection or colonization with *methicillin-resistant S. aureus (MRSA)* or *Pseudomonas species*, treatment should be with vancomycin or clindamycin or antipseudomonal antibiotic, respectively (Figure 2). Concomitant antifungal prophylaxis should be prescribed to mitigate the risk of fungal peritonitis. The duration of antibiotic therapy for an exit site infection should be modified based on the swab culture, clinical response, and in vitro susceptibility results. In case of good clinical response on the 7th day of the treatment, it could be shortened to 7-10 days instead of a 2-week antibiotic course.

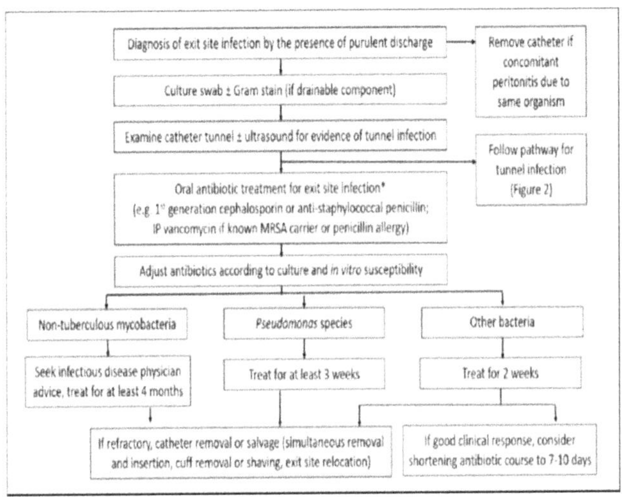


**Figure 2.** ISPD 2023 algorithm for management of PD exit-site infection

The duration of treatment of *Pseudomonas* exit site infection should be at least 3 weeks, and in case of unsatisfactory treatment response, a second antipseudomonal drug should be added. In the case of *S. aureus* infection with slow response, oral rifampicin could be considered but should never be given as monotherapy. Non-tuberculous mycobacteria (NTM) should be suspected in patients with refractory exit site infection. In that case, an examination for acid-fast bacilli by Ziehl–Neelsen staining and culture on specific media should be obtained. Although there is no standardized recommendation, treatment with two agents with in vitro activity against the clinical isolate for a minimum of 4 months is needed for NTM infection

Any tunnel infection should be treated at least 3 weeks with effective antibiotics (Figure 3). The Ultrasound examination of the tunnel might be used in the evaluation of clinical response and to guide the need for catheter removal.

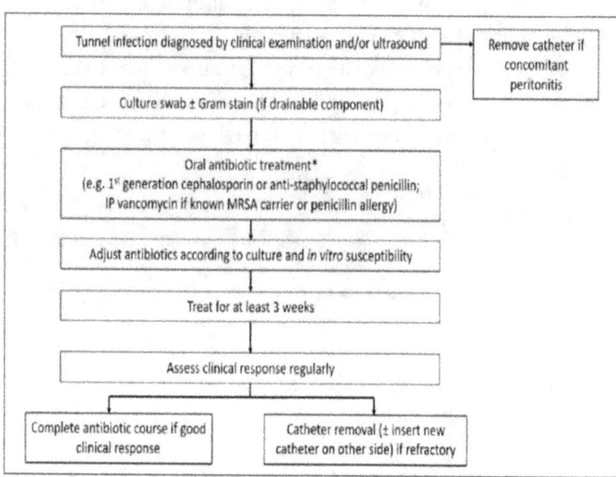


**Figure 3.** ISPD 2023 algorithm for management of PD catheter tunnel infection

When a catheter infection coexists with peritonitis, catheter removal with temporary hemodialysis treatment was advised. The reinsertion of the PD catheter should not be attempted at least 2 weeks after catheter removal, and complete resolution of peritonitis. For infection of the catheter alone, simultaneous removal and reinsertion of the catheter with a new exit site under antibiotic cover might be a rational option. The simultaneous catheter removal and reinsertion should be avoided in a case of peritonitis and/or tunnel infection caused by *P. aeruginosa*, NTM infection, and deep Dacron cuff involvement of concurrent peritonitis. In patients with extrusion of the external cuff and concomitant refractory exit-site infection, cuff shaving or removal of the external cuff should be considered. Relocation of the exit site of the catheter provided satisfactory results for patients with refractory exit site infection.

**Prevention of catheter-related infections**

- Prophylactic antibiotics should be administered immediately before catheter insertion for prevention of peritonitis. The patients should be screened for nasal S. aureus carriers and treated with nasal antibiotics.
- The exit site dressing should be left intact for 7 days after PD catheter insertion.
- The proper training and retraining programs might reduce the rate of catheter-related infection.
- Daily topical application of antibiotic cream or ointment (mupirocin or gentamicin) to the catheter exit site to prevent catheter-related infection.
- The exit site should be cleansed at least twice weekly and every time after a shower or vigorous exercise.

## References


1. Boudville N, Johnson DW, Zhao J, Bieber BA, Pisoni RL, Piraino B et al. Regional variation in the treatment and prevention of peritoneal dialysis-related infections in the Peritoneal Dialysis Outcomes and Practice Patterns Study. Nephrol Dial Transplant. 2019 Dec 1;34(12):2118-2126.
2. Perl J, Fuller DS, Bieber BA, Boudville N, Kanjanabuch T, Ito Y et al. Peritoneal Dialysis-Related Infection Rates and Outcomes: Results From the Peritoneal Dialysis Outcomes and Practice Patterns Study (PDOPPS). Am J Kidney Dis. 2020 Jul;76(1):42-53.
3. Bello AK, Okpechi IG, Osman MA, Cho Y, Cullis B, Htay H, et al. Epidemiology of peritoneal dialysis outcomes. Nat Rev Nephrol. 2022 Dec;18(12):779-793.
4. Salzer WL. Peritoneal dialysis-related peritonitis: challenges and solutions. Int J Nephrol Renovasc Dis. 2018 Jun 11;11:173-186.
5. Li PK, Chow KM, Cho Y, Fan S, Figueiredo AE, Harris T, et al. ISPD peritonitis guideline recommendations: 2022 update on prevention and treatment. Perit Dial Int. 2022 Mar;42(2):110-153.
6. Bhave G, Golper TA. ISPD 2022 recommendations for identification of causative organisms in peritonitis. Perit Dial Int. 2022 Nov;42(6):652-653.
7. Chow KM, Li PK, Cho Y, Abu-Alfa A, Bavanandan S, Brown EA et al. ISPD Catheter-related Infection Recommendations: 2023 Update. Perit Dial Int. 2023 May;43(3):201-219.
8. Khan SF. Updates on Infectious and Other Complications in Peritoneal Dialysis: Core Curriculum 2023. Am J Kidney Dis. 2023 Oct;82(4):481-490.

*Chapter 11*
*Management of anemia and mineral bone disorders in patients on*
*peritoneal dialysis*

## 11.1. Management of anemia in patients on PD

Renal anemia is defined as a low level of hemoglobin (Hb) < 12 g/dL in women and Hb <13 g/dL in men in patients with chronic kidney disease (CKD). Anemia is a frequent complication of CKD, might begin in the early stages of CKD, and could worsen with the decreasing of renal function. Renal anemia is normocytic, normochromic, and hyperproliferative, with complex and multifactorial etiology. Low production of erythropoietin (EPO) in the kidney is an important but not the only factor in the development of renal anemia. Other factors, such as decreased bone marrow response to EPO, impaired iron absorption, absolute iron deficiency, systemic inflammation with high hepcidin level, hemolysis, nutritional deficiency, and shortened survival of red blood cells could also contribute to the development of anemia in patients with CKD. KDIGO (Kidney Disease: Improving Global Outcomes) recommended the following tests for initial evaluation of anemia in patients with CKD (regardless of age and CKD stage): complete blood count (CBC), absolute reticulocyte count, serum ferritin level, serum transferrin saturation (TSAT), serum vitamin B12, and folate levels. The presence of anemia in CKD patients was associated with cognitive and sexual dysfunction, reduced exercise tolerance, left cardiac ventricular hypertrophy, and a higher incidence of cardiovascular morbidity and mortality.

Renal anemia is treated with erythropoiesis-stimulating agents (ESA). ESA are divided into shorter-acting and longer-acting agents. Epoetin alfa and epoetin beta are shorter-acting agents. The longer-acting agents are darbepoetin alfa, with a half-life of approximately 2 to 3 times longer than epoetin alfa, and methoxy polyethylene glycol-epoetin beta with a serum half-life of 130 hours. Before starting with ESA treatment, iron deficiency, vitamin B12, folic acid deficiency, occult bleeding, and other causes of anemia should be excluded. If the patient has iron deficiency (TSAT $\leq$ 30% and ferritin < 500 ng/ml (500 mg/l)), the treatment of the anemia should be started with iron supplementation. The route of iron administration should be based on the severity of iron deficiency, availability of venous access, response to prior oral iron therapy, side effects with prior oral or IV iron therapy, patient compliance, and cost. Patients who received IV iron therapy achieved target Hb levels more quickly compared to treatment with oral iron. The subsequent iron administration in CKD patients should be guided based on Hb responses to recent iron therapy, as well as ongoing blood losses, iron status tests (TSAT and ferritin), and Hb concentration.

KDIGO suggested that for adult patients on dialysis (including PD patients), the ESA therapy should be started when the hemoglobin level is between 9.0–10.0 g/dl. ESA should not be used to maintain Hb concentration above 11.5 g/dl in adult patients on dialysis. Subcutaneous administration of ESA is the preferred route of administration for PD patients. The Hb concentration should be measured at least monthly in dialysis patients during the treatment with ESA. The red cell transfusions in dialysis patients are indicated when ESA therapy is ineffective (hemoglobinopathies, bone marrow failure, ESA resistance), and when the risks of ESA therapy might outweigh its benefits (previous or current malignancy, previous stroke). KDIGO recommends avoiding, when possible, red cell transfusions to minimize the general risks related to their use, especially in patients eligible for organ transplantation, to minimize the risk of allosensitization.

The hypoxia-inducible factor prolyl hydroxylase inhibitor (HIF-PHI) [roxadustat, daprodustat, vadadustat, molidustat, and enarodustat] is a new class of oral drugs for the treatment of renal anemia. The HIF-PHI inhibits degradation of factor hypoxia-inducible factor alpha (HIF-$\alpha$). HIF-$\alpha$ translocates to the cell nucleus to bind with hypoxia-inducible factor beta (HIF-$\beta$) to promote the transcription of the erythropoietin gene for higher EPO production with improved iron metabolism. A few recent studies with patients on PD demonstrated that roxadustat, vadadustat, and daprodustat were effective in correcting or maintaining hemoglobin levels within the target range.

## 11.2. Management of mineral bone disorders in patients on PD

Chronic kidney disease-mineral bone disorder (CKD-MBD) is a common systemic condition in patients with CKD that causes bone abnormalities and ectopic calcification. The Kidney Disease: Improving Global Outcomes (KDIGO) defined CKD-MBD as the presence of one or combination of the following parameters: laboratory abnormalities of calcium (Ca), inorganic phosphorus (P), parathyroid hormone (PTH) or vitamin D; bone abnormalities in turnover, mineralization, volume, linear growth or strength, and calcification of the vasculature or other soft tissues. The imbalance of calcium-phosphorus metabolism could cause heart valve and vascular calcification which has been identified as major risk factor for cardiovascular morbidity and mortality in patients with CKD. The large prospective multicenter study in the Netherlands included 586 patients on PD and 1043 patients on HD (1997-2004). The elevated plasma phosphorus and Ca x P concentrations were associated with increased cardiovascular mortality risk in PD and HD patients.

The CKD-MBD complex consists from six types of bone disorders: hyperparathyroid bone disease, mixed bone disease, osteomalacia, adynamic bone disease (ABD), amyloid bone disease, and aluminum bone disease. The most prevalent pattern in HD patients is secondary hyperparathyroidism. The PD patients had a higher incidence of adynamic bone disease (Table 1).

**Table 1:** Prevalence of CKD-MBD determined by bone biopsy in PD and HD patients

|  | PD | HD |
|---|---|---|
| Adynamic bone disease | 50% | 19% |
| Mild disease | 20% | 3% |
| Hyperparathyroid bone disease | 18% | 34% |
| Mixed bone disease | 5% | 32% |
| Osteomalacia | 5% | 10% |
| Normal bone histology | 2% | 2% |

(Rroji M et al. The Bone and Mineral Disorder in Patients Undergoing Chronic PD. Evolving Strategies in PD. InTech; 2018.)

Numerous specific factors have been implicated in the pathophysiology of adynamic bone disease in peritoneal dialysis, including:

**Accumulation of advanced glycation end products (AGEs):** PD patients, due to dextrose-based PD solutions, are prone to have higher glucose levels which ultimately inhibit bone mineralization by preventing calcium uptake in bone cells.

**High levels of calcium and magnesium found in dialysate:** high magnesium and calcium concentrations in serum might inhibit parathyroid hormone secretion.

**High levels of sclerostin:** sclerostin is a glycoprotein produced by osteocytes, and inhibits proliferation and differentiation of osteoclasts leading to low bone turn over.

**Low levels of serum albumin:** Hypoalbuminemia caused by malnutrition and/or loss through the peritoneal membrane was associated with reduced level of PTH and development of ABD.

Adynamic bone disease in PD patients could be prevented with the usage of peritoneal dialysis fluid with low-calcium (2.5 mEq/L). Moraes et al. managed to reduce the inhibition of parathyroid hormone secretion and development of ABD in PD patients with switching from high (3.5 mEq/L) to low-calcium (2.5 mEq/L) peritoneal dialysis fluid.

Serum accumulation of the phosphorus is increasing with the deterioration of the chronic kidney disease. High phosphorus level stimulates the secretion of PTH with monoclonal nodular hyperplasia of the parathyroid glands (secondary hyperparathyroidism), decreases levels of calcium-sensing receptor and vitamin D receptor, decreases activity of 1-alpha-hydroxylase enzyme with low serum $1,25(OH)_2D_3$ levels. Serum phosphate excess was an independent risk factor for death in dialysis patients because of the association with the endothelial dysfunction, increased fibroblast growth factor 23 (FGF-23), and left ventricular hypertrophy. FGF23 is a circulating peptide secreted by bone osteocytes and osteoblasts as a response to calcitriol, increased dietary phosphate load, PTH, and calcium. The primary function of FGF23 is to maintain normal serum phosphate concentration. In CKD patients, increased FGF23 levels were associated with the increased risk of cardiovascular diseases and mortality. The dialytic removal of phosphorus is limited compared to the removal of phosphorus with residual renal function (diuresis). Limitation in dietary phosphate intake and the use of phosphate binder is necessary to maintain a normal serum phosphorus level in dialysis patients with declining residual renal function. The calcium-containing phosphate binders are available as calcium carbonate and calcium acetate. Calcium salts should be administered carefully, because they could raise serum calcium levels especially when are used together with vitamin D and high calcium dialyzing solutions, leading to PTH suppression, ABD, vascular calcifications and increased cardiovascular mortality. Sevelamer, lanthanum carbonate, and sucroferric oxyhydroxide are calcium-free phosphate binders developed for management of hyperphosphatemia in dialysis patients with normal or high serum levels of calcium. The use of sevelamer was associated with more frequent occurrence of diarrhea or constipation in PD patients and slightly increased risk of peritonitis caused by Gram-negative microorganisms. Iron-based phosphate binders (sucroferric oxyhydroxide) are novel and promising drugs.

Due to the peritoneal loss of 25 (OH) vitamin D and the precursor of active vitamin D during PD, the patients have high risk of developing vitamin D deficiency. The decline in renal mass in CKD patients and hyperphosphatemia with increased FGF23 levels suppress the renal synthesis of calcitriol. Low calcitriol concentrations increase PTH secretion from parathyroid glands. The correction of vitamin D in CKD patients should be started either with cholecalciferol or calcifediol (800–1000 UI/day). Calcitriol or paricalcitol should be added only when the PTH levels are stable at 450–

500 pg/mL in the absence of high serum calcium and/or phosphorus levels. Cinacalcet acts directly upon the parathyroid cell calcium-sensing receptor (CaR) and suppress PTH secretion without increasing serum calcium and phosphate levels. Portoles et al. showed that the addition of cinacalcet to conventional treatment in PD patients with resistant hyperparathyroidism has improved the achievement of targets recommended by KDIGO.

The serum levels of calcium in PD patients depend from dietary calcium intake, calcium supplement dose, intake of vitamin D analogs, and influx of calcium from high-calcium PD dialysate. In individuals with CKD, both hypocalcemia and hypercalcemia were associated with higher mortality rates. Serum calcium levels were associated with suppression (high calcium) or stimulation (low calcium) of PTH secretion and bone remodeling process. KDIGO 2017 recommended the use of a dialysate calcium concentration between 1.25 and 1.50 mmol/l (2.5 and 3.0 mEq/l) in PD and HD patients.

The prevention and treatment of CKD-MBD in PD patients should be done with:

- Measurement of serum calcium and phosphate every 1–3 months, PTH every 3–6 months, and alkaline phosphatase activity every 12 months or more frequently in the presence of elevated PTH. 25(OH)D (calcidiol) levels might be measured, and repeated testing determined by baseline values and therapeutic interventions.
- BMD testing (densitometry) might be performed to assess fracture risk if results will impact treatment decisions in patients with CKD stage 5 and evidence of CKD-MBD and/or risk factors for osteoporosis. Bone biopsy could be performed if the knowledge of the type of renal osteodystrophy will impact on the treatment decisions.
- Serum markers of bone resorption (TRAP5b, s-NTX, s-CTX, s-ICTP or CTX-MMP) and bone formation (s-PINP, AF, s-PICP) should not be routinely measured.
- FGF23 may be a more stable marker of phosphate metabolism in dialysis patients compared to PTH or serum phosphate. A single measurement of FGF23 could more precisely determine the phosphate metabolism issue.
- Determination of the presence of vascular and valvular calcifications with radiodiagnostic imaging.

**References**

1. Kidney Disease: Improving Global Outcomes (KDIGO) Anemia Work Group. KDIGO Clinical Practice Guideline for Anemia in Chronic Kidney Disease. Kidney inter., Suppl. 2012; 2: 279–335.
2. Wetmore JB, Peng Y, Monda KL, Kats AM, Kim DH, Bradbury BD et al. Trends in anemia management practices in patients receiving hemodialysis and peritoneal dialysis: a retrospective cohort analysis. Am J Nephrol. 2015;41(4-5):354-61.
3. Perlman RL, Zhao J, Fuller DS. International Anemia Prevalence and Management in Peritoneal Dialysis Patients. Peritoneal Dialysis International. 2019;39(6):539-546.
4. Li PKT, Choy ASM, Bavanandan S, Chen W, Foo M, Kanjanabuch T et al. Anemia Management in Peritoneal Dialysis: Perspectives From the Asia Pacific Region. Kidney Med. 2021 Apr 20;3(3):405-411.
5. Del Vecchio L, Cavalli A, Locatelli F. Anemia management in patients on peritoneal dialysis. Contrib Nephrol. 2012;178:89-94.
6. Peritoneal Dialysis Anemia Management Protocol. BC Renal.
7. Marajah, Kenisha, "Anemia Management for Patients Receiving Peritoneal Dialysis" (2018). Doctor of Nursing Practice. https://athenaeum.uiw.edu/uiw _dnp/49.
8. Li J, Haase VH, Hao CM. Updates on Hypoxia-Inducible Factor Prolyl Hydroxylase Inhibitors in the Treatment of Renal Anemia. Kidney Dis (Basel). 2022 Oct 31;9(1):1-11.
9. Moraes TP, Bucharles SG, Ribeiro SC. Low-calcium peritoneal dialysis solution is effective in bringing PTH levels to the range recommended by current guidelines in patients with PTH levels < 150 pg/dL. Jornal Brasileiro de Nefrologia. 2010;32(3):275-280.
10. Noordzij M, Korevaar JC, Bos WJ, Boeschoten EW, Dekker FW, Bossuyt PM et al. Mineral metabolism and cardiovascular morbidity and mortality risk: peritoneal dialysis patients compared with haemodialysis patients. Nephrol Dial Transplant. 2006;21:2513–2520.
11. Kidney Disease: Improving Global Outcomes (KDIGO) CKD-MBD Update Work Group. KDIGO 2017 Clinical Practice Guideline Update for the Diagnosis, Evaluation, Prevention, and Treatment of Chronic Kidney Disease–Mineral and Bone Disorder (CKD-MBD). Kidney Int Suppl. 2017;7:1–59.
12. Rroji, M., Spahia, N., Barbullushi, M., & Seferi, S. (2018). The Bone and Mineral Disorder in Patients Undergoing Chronic Peritoneal Dialysis. InTech.

13.Nitta, K., Hanafusa, N. & Tsuchiya, K. Mineral bone disorders (MBD) in patients on peritoneal dialysis. Ren Replace Ther 5, 4 (2019). https://doi.org/10.1186/s41100-019-0200-4

*Chapter 12*
*Nutrition in patients on peritoneal dialysis*

Adequate nutrition in patients on peritoneal dialysis has a significant impact on the quality of life and survival of the patients. The assessment and correction of nutritional habits in PD patients might be challenging and usually requires an approach by a multidisciplinary team guided by the renal dietician. The team should evaluate the health condition, nutritional status, and nutritional habits of the patient and to ensure continuous education of the patient with adequate protein and energy intake. All PD guidelines recommend regular assessment of patient nutritional status: dry body weight, appetite, dietary intake, and laboratory markers of nutrition (albumin, cholesterol, potassium, phosphate, and bicarbonate).

Malnutrition is defined as an imbalance between the supply of the body with nutrients and energy and the body's demand for them to ensure growth, maintenance, and specific functions. Compared to hemodialysis, patients on PD are particularly susceptible to malnutrition, and it is believed that 30–50% of these patients are malnourished. Moreover, PD patients often exhibit a particular profile of malnutrition with decreased protein stores: protein-energy wasting (PEW) with persistence of overweight and obesity. PEW is an important risk factor for morbidity and mortality in PD patients. A cohort study of 555 PD patients reported that the prevalence of PEW in PD patients was 27.3%, and 196 deaths were observed during the mean follow-up of 25.5 months. The study revealed that the presence of PEW was not significantly associated with a higher risk of death after adjusting for potential confounders. However, the individual PEW criteria of decreased serum albumin level and low muscle mass were found to be independent predictors of all-cause mortality in the multivariable analysis of patients receiving PD.

## 12.1. Protein-Energy Wasting (PEW): diagnosis, pathophysiology, and clinical significance

The criteria for diagnosis of PEW proposed by the International Society for Renal Nutrition and Metabolism (ISRNM) are:

- Serum chemistry: serum albumin < 3.8 g/100ml, serum prealbumin < 3.0 g/200ml, serum cholesterol < 100 mg/100ml.

91

- Body Mass Index: BMI < 23 kg/m$^2$. Unintentional weight loss: 5% over 3 months or 10% over 6 months, total body fat percentage < 10%.
- Muscle Mass: muscle wasting (5% reduced muscle mass over 3 months or 10% over 6 months); Reduced mid-arm circumference (>10% reduction in relation to 50th percentile of reference population).
- Dietary Intake: unintentionally low dietary protein intake (DPI) < 0.8 g/kg/day and/or dietary energy intake (DEI) < 25 kcal/kg/day for at least two months.

Protein-energy wasting in PD patients is developed by the loss of the serum amino acids into the peritoneal dialysate (approximately 8 to 12 g of protein and 6–8 g of albumin each day). High transporters are particularly susceptible to protein loss. Peritonitis could also lead to increased permeability of the peritoneal membrane with additional loss of proteins. The glucose absorbed in the serum from the peritoneal dialysate has an important role in body fat accumulation. For example, absorption of 100 to 200 g glucose from dialysate provides an additional 400 to 800 kcal per day. PD patients are prone to increasing fat stores in the body in the first two years of dialysis, while muscle stores are decreasing. The loss of protein during peritoneal dialysis is not the only factor associated with PEW. Inflammation, chronic kidney disease, metabolic acidosis, inadequate dialysis, inadequate nutrient intake, comorbid conditions, psychosocial factors, and physical inactivity are also factors associated with PEW (Figure 1).

Inflammation plays a key role in the pathogenesis of PEW and also accelerates atherosclerosis and arteriosclerosis. Malnutrition, inflammation, and atherosclerosis (MIA) syndrome have been associated with high rates of cardiovascular morbidity and mortality in PD patients. De Mutsert R et al. found that the 2-year mortality rate increased by up to 70% in patients who had MIA syndrome compared with a mortality rate of 10% or less in patients who had no MIA syndrome.

Inadequate nutritional intake is another important factor in the development of PEW. The Kidney Dialysis Outcomes Quality Initiative (KDOQI) guidelines recommend a daily energy intake of 35 kcal/kg for patients on peritoneal dialysis with age under 60 years, and 30–35 kcal/kg for patients with age over 60 years. The daily protein intake should be of 1.2–1.3 g/kg for PD patients. Studies have shown that only small minority of PD patients managed to consume this amount of calories and protein. Continuous serum absorption of glucose from peritoneal dialysis solutions and abdominal fullness induced by the dialysate, suppress the appetite and lead to low caloric intake.

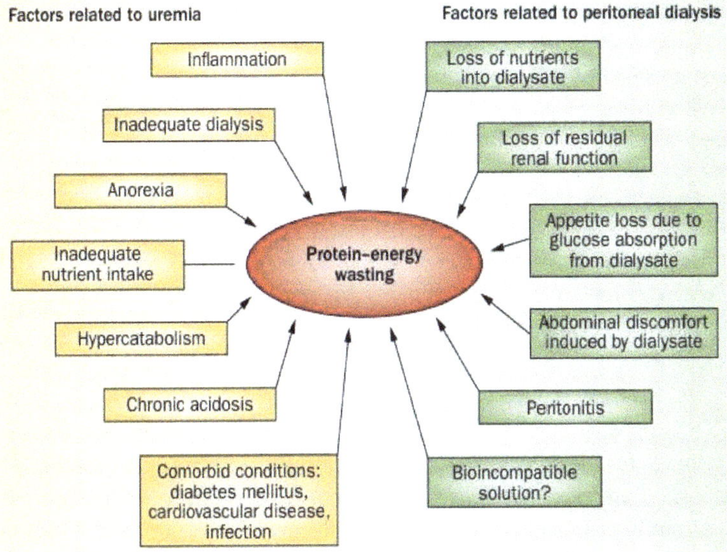



**Figure 1.** Factors associated with PEW in patients on peritoneal dialysis. (Han SH.et al. Nutrition in patients on peritoneal dialysis. Nat Rev Nephrol. 2012(8): 163–175)

Patients who are malnourished are prone to exacerbation of pre-existing comorbidities including cardiovascular diseases, sexual dysfunction, anemia, and sarcopenia. Dong et al. showed that PD patients with daily protein intake (DPI) of < 0.73 g/kg had worse outcomes, but when a DPI of > 0.94 g/kg was achieved, the patients experienced better outcomes and fewer complications such as peritonitis. The PEW was associated with the rate of infections in PD patients. Namely, low DPI and PEW led to frequent episodes of peritonitis with increased loss of proteins in dialysate, suppressed appetite (related to the release of IL-1 during the acute phase response), and energy loss. Elevated levels of the C-reactive protein (CRP) directly correlated with malnutrition and mortality in patients.

## 12.2. Prevention and treatment of PEW

Treatment of PEW in patients on peritoneal dialysis requires a multidisciplinary approach with careful nutritional assessment, dietary counseling, and proper nutritional support.

General approach:

- Measurements for monitoring the nutritional status of patients on peritoneal dialysis (Table 1);
- Treatment of comorbid or catabolic conditions;
- Dietary counseling: dietary counseling might be useful if inadequate nutritional intake is a cause of PEW (Table 2);
- Oral appetite stimulants: Megestrol acetate tablets increase appetite via stimulation of neuropeptide Y in the hypothalamus. A few small studies showed positive effects of the administration of Megestrol acetate on the improvement of nutritional status in PD patients. However, larger randomized studies are needed to confirm the efficiency;
- Oral nutritional supplements: oral nutritional supplements provide energy and biological value proteins and might be beneficial for elderly patients with PEW on chronic PD.

Peritoneal dialysis-related approach:

- Preserve residual kidney function (RKF): the decrease in RKF is associated with lower clearance of middle molecules, increased systemic inflammation, and PEW;
- Maintain optimal fluid balance;
- Maintain adequate dialysis dose: the dialysis dose should be increased to improve dialysis adequacy in PD patients who are suspected to be subdialysed accompanied with anorexia and inadequate nutritional intake;
- Correct acidosis: acidosis leads to proteolysis of muscles mediated via the ubiquitin-proteasome system, as well as a decrease in albumin synthesis, and reduced expression of IGF-I and growth hormone. Correction of acidosis led to improvement in patients' nutritional status. The bicarbonate-buffered peritoneal dialysis solution showed the most favorable outcomes. Also, therapy with oral sodium bicarbonate successfully improves plasma levels of bicarbonate. KDOQI guidelines recommend the therapeutic target of bicarbonate levels of $\geq$ 22 mmol/l in patients with kidney failure on PD;

- Use of amino acid-based solutions: The conventional glucose-based solutions lead to a loss of 9–12 g of proteins per day into the dialysate fluid. The use of amino acid solution could compensate for these losses and meet the nutritional requirements of patients on peritoneal dialysis.
- Use of biocompatible solutions;
- Prevent and treat peritonitis: Peritonitis increases the permeability of the peritoneal membrane and loss of proteins in dialysate solution.

**Table 1.** Recommended measurements for monitoring nutritional status of patients on peritoneal dialysis

| Category | Measure | Frequency |
|---|---|---|
| I. Measurements that should be performed routinely in all patients | serum level of albumin, | Monthly |
| | % of usual post-drain  body weight | Monthly |
| | % of standard body weight | every 6 months |
| | triceps skinfold thicknesses | every 6 months |
| | arm circumference | every 6 months |
| | dietary interview and/or diary | every 6 months |
| | protein equivalent of nitrogen appearance or protein catabolic ratio (PCR) | every 4 months |
| II. Measurements that could be used to extend the measurements obtained in category I. | body composition assessed by the sum of the 4 skinfold thicknesses (biceps, triceps, subscapular, suprailiac) | as needed |
| | hand-grip strength | as needed |
| | waist circumference | as needed |
| III. Laboratory parameters, if they are low, there is a need for a more rigorous examination of the nutritional status | serum level of creatinine<br><br>serum level of  urea<br><br>serum level of cholesterol | every 6 months |

(Maria Avesani C et al.  Nutritional Aspects of Adult Patients Treated With Chronic Peritoneal Dialysis. J Bras Nefrol. 2006; 28(4): 232-238.)

**Table 2.** Recommended nutritional intakes for PD patients – summary

| Nutrients | Recommended intakes per day |
|---|---|
| Energy | 35 kcal/kg/ per day in patients < 60 years<br><br>30-35 kcal/kg/ per day in patients > 60 years |
| Protein | KDIGO: 1.2–1.3 g/kg/per day<br><br>(at least 50% of high biological value) |
| Fats | 30% of total energy supply |
| Water and fluids | as per residual diuresis |
| Potassium | the standard recommendation is 3500 to 4500 milligrams daily |
| Calcium | individualized, usually 1000-1200 mg per day |
| Phosphorous | 800-1000 mg/day (adjusted to higher protein needs) when serum phosphorous is > 5.5 mg/dl (1.78 mmol/l) |
| Sodium | 2000-3000 mg |

(Council on Renal Nutrition, Nutrition and Peritoneal Dialysis. Available online: https://www.kidn ey.org/atoz/content/nutripd)

# References


1. Kittiskulnam P, Chuengsaman P, Kanjanabuch T, Katesomboon S, Tungsanga S, Tiskajornsiri K et al. Protein-Energy Wasting and Mortality Risk Prediction Among Peritoneal Dialysis Patients. Journal of Renal Nutrition. 2021; 31(6): 679-686.

2. Mehrotra R, Duong U, Jiwakanon S, P. Kovesdy C, Moran J, D. Kopple J et al. Serum Albumin as a Predictor of Mortality in Peritoneal Dialysis: Comparisons With Hemodialysis. American Journal of Kidney Diseases. 2011; 58(3):418-428.

3. Kim, SM., Kang, M., Kang, E. *et al.* Associations among body composition parameters and quality of life in peritoneal dialysis patients. *Sci Rep* **12**, 19192 (2022). https://doi.org/10.1038/s 41598-022-19715-2

4. Schaible UE, Kaufmann SHE. Malnutrition and Infection: Complex Mechanisms and Global Impacts. PLoS Med. 2007;4(5):e115.

5. Han SH, Han DS. Nutrition in patients on peritoneal dialysis. Nat Rev Nephrol. 2012; 8:163–175.

6. Kiebalo T, Holotka J, Habura I, Pawlaczyk K. Nutritional Status in Peritoneal Dialysis: Nutritional Guidelines, Adequacy and the Management of Malnutrition. Nutrients. 2020 Jun 8;12(6):1715.

7. Maria Avesani C, Heimbürger O, Stenvinkel P, Lindholm B. Nutritional Aspects of Adult Patients Treated With Chronic Peritoneal Dialysis. J Bras Nefrol. 2006; 28(4): 232-238.

8. Council on Renal Nutrition, Nutrition and Peritoneal Dialysis. Available online: https://www.kidney.org/atoz/content/nutripd.

9. Fouque D, Kalantar-Zadeh K, Kopple J, Cano N, Chauveau P, Cuppari L et al. A proposed nomenclature and diagnostic criteria for protein-energy wasting in acute and chronic kidney disease. Kidney Int. 2008 Feb;73(4):391-398.

*Chapter 13*
## *Survival and health-related quality of life in PD patients*

The World Health Organization defined the health-related quality of life (HrQOL) as a "complete state of physical, mental and social well-being and not merely the absence of disease and infirmity". It is an important factor in the evaluation of health status in patients on kidney replacement therapy (KRT). HrQOL had a significant impact on the morbidity and mortality of the patients on the KRT. These patients are with chronic kidney disease, many additional comorbidities, and treatment-related complications, which often lead to immobility, cognitive dysfunction, sleep disturbances, depression, sexual dysfunction, and anxiety. The assessment of HrQOL in CKD patients is complex and there is no gold standard instrument (Table 1).

**Table 1.** HrQOL instruments for the CKD population

| Questionnaire | Characteristics |
|---|---|
| Karnofsky Performance Status Score | Measure the level of patient activity and medical requirements |
| Sickness impact profile | Measure sickness-related dysfunction in patients' daily activities |
| Short-Form-36 (SF-36) | The most commonly used.<br><br>Multi-item scale that evaluate limitations in physical, social and usual role activities due to health or emotional problems. It also assessed the general mental status, body pain, vitality, and general health perception. |
| Kidney Disease Questionnaire | Disease-specific questionnaire.<br><br>Include 5 dimensions: physical symptoms, fatigue, depression, relationships with others and frustrations. |
| Kidney Disease QOL, KDQOF-36 | Similar to SF-36, supplemented with kidney disease and dialysis-related problems. |

Patients with chronic kidney disease, regardless of the type of KRT, had worse HrQOL than the age-matched controls from the general population. Many studies showed that in all age groups, dialysis (HD or PD) was associated with lower HrQOL compared to kidney transplantation. When comparing HD and PD, the results are ambiguous and uncertain. The study by Turkmen K et al. involved 90 HD patients and 64 PD patients receiving KRT for at least 3 months who were screened for the assessment of sleep quality (SQ), HrQOL, and depression. Physical and mental component scales of HrQOL were significantly higher (better scores) in HD patients compared to PD patients (P = 0.001). Significantly more PD patients were with depression when compared to HD patients (P=0.001). Independent predictors of depression were the mental component scale of HrQOL, gender (female), and dialysis modality (PD).

The most comprehensive comparison of HrQOL between PD and HD was a meta-analysis performed by Queeley GL et al. The analysis included a total of 4318 patients from 15 different studies. The majority of the studies favored peritoneal dialysis over hemodialysis as a more effective dialysis modality in all 3 analyzed domains: general, physical-functioning, and psychological-functioning domains. The results did not confirm that peritoneal dialysis was more effective in the 3 analyzed domains compared to hemodialysis.

The United States Renal Data System (USRDS) showed that during the last decade, patient survival, especially survival in the initial year on dialysis had improved markedly in PD compared to HD patients. It is less certain if the better survival of PD patients was followed by improved HrQOL.

The study by Guney I et al. included 20 APD and 48 CAPD patients who were compared in terms of sleep quality, HrQOL, and depression. HrQOL and depression were evaluated by the Short Form of Medical Outcomes Study and Beck Depression Inventory, respectively. Moderate or severe sleep problems were found in 60% and 69% of the APD and CAPD patients, respectively, with no significant difference. The mean physical component score was $51.1 \pm 21.2$ and $48.9 \pm 18.2$ in APD and CAPD patients, respectively, with no significant difference. The mean mental component score was $47.5 \pm 20.1$ in APD patients and $42.4 \pm 19.5$ in CAPD patients, with no significant difference. Depression was detected in 70% of APD and in 62.5% of CAPD patients, with no significant difference. This study showed that sleep quality, HrQOL, and depression were similar in APD and CAPD patients.

**Table 2.** Factors associated with HrQOL in PD patients (summary)

| Factors associated to HrQOL | Explanation |
| --- | --- |
| Age | HrQOL scores are lower in elderly patients, mainly due to physical impairment |
| Gender | Changes in the hypothalamic-pituitary-gonadal axis make women more prone to sleep disorders, depression, and cognitive dysfunction |
| Ethnicity | Conflicting results from different studies (lower HrQOL in Indo-Asians than in Europeans) |
| Socioeconomic status | High social support was associated with better HrQOL and a lower risk of hospitalization. However, HrQOL was not influenced by education level and income. |
| Spirituality | Religious dimensions of spirituality had a positive impact on quality of life. |
| Health literacy | Personal ability to cope effectively with health information is associated with better outcomes. |
| Comorbidities | Diabetes mellitus and cardiovascular diseases had negative impact. |
| Depression and anxiety | In PD patients, depression is related to poor outcome, higher rates of peritonitis, frequent hospitalization, and sleep disturbances. |
| Anemia | Negative influence on HrQOL |
| GFR and residual renal function | Higher residual renal function is associated with better HrQOL |
| Gastrointestinal tract (GIT) | PD patients more frequently have GIT problems. The inflamed gut barrier enables translocation of intestinal bacteria and peritonitis. |
| Sexual dysfunction | In both sexes is associated with poorer HrQOL |

| | |
|---|---|
| Nutritional status | Protein-energy wasting (PEW) and malnutrition are associated with cardiovascular diseases and mortality. |
| Infection/Inflammatory status | Inverse correlation between CRP and HrQOL. Inverse correlation between rate of peritonitis and HrQOL. |
| Sleep | Sleep disorders are associated with lower HrQOL and higher mortality risk. |
| Dialysis vintage | Inverse correlation |
| CAPD vs APD | CAPD: less sleep interruptions<br><br>APD: less peritonitis, fewer hernias, more freedom |
| Adequacy | Uncertain effects on HrQOL |
| PD solutions | The use of a biocompatible solution with neutral pH and low concentration of glucose-degradation products provides better residual renal function and less peritonitis. |

(Aguiar R et al. Health-related quality of life in peritoneal dialysis patients: A narrative review. Semin Dial. 2019 Sep;32(5):452-462.)

The low HrQOL in PD patients was associated with an increased rate of hospital admissions and higher mortality. The identification of the factors that influence HrQOL is crucial for the better survival of PD patients. Strategies that include nurse-led management programs, telephone follow-up especially during the initial period of PD, and high levels of exercise training and regular psychological support programs could improve patients' quality satisfaction and quality of life.

# References


1. Aguiar R, Pei M, Qureshi AR, Lindholm B. Health-related quality of life in peritoneal dialysis patients: A narrative review. Semin Dial. 2019 Sep;32(5):452-462.
2. Queeley GL, Campbell ES. Comparing Treatment Modalities for End-Stage Renal Disease: A Meta-Analysis. Am Health Drug Benefits. 2018 May;11(3):118-127.
3. Turkmen K, Yazici R, Solak Y, Guney I, Altintepe L, Yeksan M, et al. Health-related quality of life, sleep quality, and depression in peritoneal dialysis and hemodialysis patients. Hemodial Int. 2012 Apr;16(2):198-206.
4. Guney I, Solak Y, Atalay H, Yazici R, Altintepe L, Kara F et al. Comparison of effects of automated peritoneal dialysis and continuous ambulatory peritoneal dialysis on health-related quality of life, sleep quality, and depression. Hemodial Int. 2010 Oct;14(4):515-22.

*Chapter 14*

*No Place Like Home!*
*The role of peritoneal dialysis in natural disasters and pandemics*

A disaster is a "state of emergency" event in which more than 10 people are killed, and more than 100 people are affected and requires a specialized national or international response. Eighteen natural and biological hazards are included in the US Federal Emergency Management Association National Risk Index. These events could destroy health care infrastructure, and loss of medical personnel, putting vulnerable populations at risk. Patients with kidney failure on hemodialysis are particularly susceptible to disasters because they depend on electricity, clean water, medical equipment, transportation, and medical staff. The lack of these resources could result in the absence of life-sustaining dialysis treatment and death of these patients.

Peritoneal dialysis (PD) is a preferred modality of kidney replacement therapy (KRT) in emergencies due to several advantages:

- The PD exchanges could be done manually with no need for electrical power and a huge amount of clean water.
- The PD patients do not need transportation to and from a dialysis facility.
- The PD patients are independent while they are performing the dialysis treatment, and they do not need medical assistance which might be lacking during natural disasters.
- The patients perform PD in their homes, so during a pandemic, the risk of disease spread among patients and healthcare workers is reduced.

Kumar V et al. described two patients who were saved with peritoneal dialysis during the devastating flash floods in Leh, India, in August 2010. More than two hundred people died, and a large number of people were rendered homeless during the disaster. The existing health care, telecommunications, and transport infrastructure were extensively damaged. The affected areas remained cut off from the rest of the world for 4 days. The first case-patient was a 30-year-old man who had been on continuous ambulatory PD (CAPD) for 7 years. The patient's house and his dialysis supplies had been lost by the flood. Fortunately, he was able to find a patient on PD in another area who had escaped the catastrophe. He continued PD using borrowed supplies and survived the disaster.

105

The second case patient was a 29-year-old Indian army soldier whose unit was engaged in relief operations. Acute gastroenteritis with profuse diarrhea caused the development of acute kidney failure in the soldier with the need for dialysis treatment. Because no HD facilities were available, the treating physician started treatment with peritoneal dialysis using a rigid catheter on a stylet. The patient survived till the evacuation and continued treatment with hemodialysis till complete recovery. The second case highlights that the knowledge of PD catheter insertion could save lives in unexpected and desperate circumstances, and should be acquired by any nephrologist.

## 14.1. Peritoneal dialysis during COVID-19 pandemic

The COVID-19 pandemic was a serious medical and social problem that challenged the health care systems in every country in the world. The patients on maintenance hemodialysis were at higher risk of developing severe COVID-19 disease, because of their compromised immunity and the underlying chronic kidney disease with co-morbidities. Peritoneal dialysis could be offered as a safer home-based modality of RRT to patients requiring chronic dialysis during pandemics as well as acute dialysis in the health care units.

## 14.2 Chronic peritoneal dialysis in COVID-19 pandemic

The 'stay-at-home' messages given during the COVID-19 pandemic put the PD as the preferred modality of RRT for patients on maintenance dialysis. The hemodialysis is performed by medical personnel in hemodialysis units with dialysis machines. Peritoneal dialysis is easily performed by patients themselves at their home, therefore can avoid in-center hospital visits, unlike patients on hemodialysis. Thus, PD patients can avoid undue exposure to the coronavirus. Medical consultations and PD prescriptions could be given by using telemedicine with the referral center, also minimizing the risk of SARS-CoV-2 infection. During a pandemic, due to an enormous number of infected patients, many hospitals were temporarily transformed into COVID-19 units. The number of healthcare workers was also reduced due to infection or quarantine.

On 28 March 2020, the International Society of Peritoneal Dialysis published its strategies regarding COVID-19 infection prevention in PD patients. The chronic PD should be continued in a room dedicated to PD procedures as before the pandemic, following the recommendations for isolation and prevention of COVID-19 infection. In cases when PD patients need support, family members are preferred before medical nurses. In the case of a positive PD patient, the PD effluent should be considered infected and must be properly disposed of. PD effluent should be disposed of by draining into the toilet and avoiding splash, with the use of adequate personal protective equipment including gloves, mask, and eye shield. Household bleach in dilution of 1:10 could be put in the toilet and left for 5 min before flushing. Used PD bags and tubings should be placed in a plastic bag, sealed, and put in another bag (double bagged) before being discarded. PET and clearance tests for the assessment of peritoneal membrane transport function in patients on peritoneal dialysis should be avoided during a pandemic. PD peritonitis could also be managed via "video consultation" and the patient should start the intraperitoneal application of antibiotics as they have been trained for that before the start of PD. Patient admission to the hospital was advised only in case of refractory peritonitis.

Ronco et al. published that PD patients had a three times lower rate of COVID-19 infection and a significantly lower rate of all-cause hospitalization compared to HD patients (2: 5 patients/month). The PD patients were coordinated through telemedicine and none of them complained about a lack of care or attention by referral center.

## 14.3 Peritoneal dialysis in COVID-19-associated acute kidney injury

Kidney injury was the second most common complication, after lung injury in COVID-19-infected patients. The incidence of acute kidney injury (AKI) varied between studies, from 5% to 29% of the infected patients within a median period of 7–14 days after hospital admission. The retrospective observational study by Fisher et al evaluated the incidence of AKI in 3345 adults with COVID-19 and 1265 without COVID-19, who were hospitalized in a large New York City health system. AKI occurred in 56.9% of patients positive for COVID-19 compared with 37.2% of those negative for COVID-19 (RR 1.5, 95% CI, 1.4 to 16). From Covid-19 positive patients with AKI, 4.9% required treatment with acute RRT compared to 1.6% Covid-19 negative patients with AKI (RR 3.1, 95% CI, 2.0 to 4.9). The modalities of used RRT were: continuous renal replacement therapy (CRRT) in 31.7%, prolonged intermittent renal replacement therapy (PIRRT) in 6.7%, PD in 9.8%, and HD in 51.8% of patients. According to recommendations, CRRT was the preferred modality, but acute PD could be also used as a modality of KRT for COVID-19 induced AKI in case of unavailability of CRRT. PD requires less equipment when compared with extracorporeal dialysis and could help to overcome the shortage of dialysis machines and healthcare workers.

The first use of acute PD for the treatment of COVID-19 induced AKI was made by Hugh Cairns in the intensive care units (ICUs) at Kings College Hospital, London, due to the shortage of CRRT. Twenty-seven patients admitted in ICU were treated with automated peritoneal dialysis (APD). The outcomes were as follows: 7 patients were with recovered kidney function, 3 patients died because of COVID-19 infection, and 17 patients remained on chronic PD. APD was the preferred modality because the cycler could be moved and installed anywhere.

Few clinical studies demonstrated that PD provided similar outcomes regarding survival and kidney function, as it was achieved by other dialysis techniques such as CRRT and HD in the treatment of AKI induced by COVID-19. Moreover, the gentle and prolonged removal of body fluids and toxins during the PD reduced the risk of hemodynamic instability in critically ill COVID-19 patients. A case series from two hospitals in New York City showed that COVID-19 patients with AKI and cardiac involvement who were treated with PD had lower mortality rate at 28 days, faster recovery of kidney function, and fewer complications from infections, compared to patients treated with CRRT. In case of compromised ventilation in patients, the use of small and frequent dwells with APD might avoid compromise in ventilation without affecting the adequacy of PD. The hypercatabolic state induced by COVID-19 infection might be improved by use of amino-acid-based PD dialysate.

In the pandemic, PD offered several advantages over HD, especially in the issue of public health and prevention of further spreading of the infection, and could be effectively and safely applied not only to stable patients with KF but also to critically ill patients with AKI requiring dialysis.

**References**

1. Ronco C, Manani SM, Giuliani A, Tantillo I, Reis T, Brown EA. Remote patient management of peritoneal dialysis during the COVID-19 pandemic. Perit Dial Int. 2020 Jul;40(4):363-367.
2. Fisher M, Neugarten J, Bellin E, Yunes M, Stahl L, Johns T.S et al. AKI in Hospitalized Patients with and without COVID-19: A Comparison Study. J. Am. Soc. Nephrol. 2020;31:2145–2157.
3. Chen TH, Wen YH, Chen CF, Tan AC, Chen YT, Chen FY et al. The advantages of peritoneal dialysis over hemodialysis during the COVID-19 pandemic. Semin Dial. 2020 Sep;33(5):369-371.Głowacka M, Lipka S, Młynarska E, Franczyk B, Rysz J. Acute Kidney Injury in COVID-19. Int J Mol Sci. 2021 Jul 28;22(15):8081.
4. Głowacka M, Lipka S, Młynarska E, Franczyk B, Rysz J. Acute Kidney Injury in COVID-19. Int J Mol Sci. 2021 Jul 28;22(15):8081.
5. Kumar V, Ramachandran R, Rathi M, Kohli HS, Sakhuja V, Jha V. Peritoneal dialysis: the great savior during disasters. Perit Dial Int. 2013 May-Jun;33(3):327-329.
6. Auguste, Bourne. (2021). The Role of Peritoneal Dialysis in Pandemics and Natural Disasters. In: Applied Peritoneal Dialysis. Springer International Publishing. pp.457-464.
7. El Shamy O, Niralee P, Mohamed Halim A, Linda Ch, Joji T, Lookstein R et al. Acute Start Peritoneal Dialysis during the COVID-19 Pandemic: Outcomes and Experiences. JASN. 2020 August;31(8):p 1680-1682. Kanjanabuch T, Pongpirul K. Peritoneal dialysis care during the COVID-19 pandemic, Thailand. Bull World Health Organ. 2022 Feb 1;100(2):155-160.
8. Kanjanabuch T, Pongpirul K. Peritoneal dialysis care during the COVID-19 pandemic, Thailand. Bull World Health Organ. 2022 Feb 1;100(2):155-160.
9. Jeloka T, Gupta A, Prasad N, Varughese S, Mahajan S, Nayak KS et al. COVID-19 Working Group of Indian Society of Nephrology. Peritoneal Dialysis Patients During COVID 19 Pandemic. Indian J Nephrol. 2020 May-Jun;30(3):171-173.
10. Mario Cozzolino. COVID-19 pandemic era: is it time to promote home dialysis and peritoneal dialysis? Clinical Kidney Journal. 2021 March.14(1):i6–i13.
11. Hua-Jun J, Hui T, Fei X, Wen-Li Ch, Jian-Bo T, Jing S et al. COVID-19 in Peritoneal Dialysis Patients. CJASN. 2021 January; 16(1):121-123.

47997CB00003B/955